TELEDERMATOLOGY

Teledermatology: A User's Guide was written to provide practical information for those individuals contemplating or planning a teledermatology program or expanding their current use of teledermatology. It focuses on the practical aspects of teledermatology implementation while providing a comprehensive treatment of the topic.

Discussions include business models and reimbursement issues, the current status of teledermatology research, the integration of teledermatology into dermatology residency training programs, ethical considerations, confidentiality issues, and the "art of teledermatology." It explores the technical aspects of teledermatology and describes the differences between live-interactive techniques and store-and-forward techniques. This book is intended to provide both novice and seasoned teledermatologists with comprehensive and practical information on teledermatology.

Many of the chapter authors are among the world experts in teledermatology and have developed successful and viable teledermatology programs. The knowledge presented here is based on the lessons they have learned in the course of teledermatology development.

DR. HON S. PAK is Director of Advanced Information Technology Group for the U.S. Army's Telemedicine and Advanced Technology Research Center (TATRC) at Fort Detrick, MD.

DR. KAREN E. EDISON is Philip C. Anderson Professor and Chairman of the Department of Dermatology, Medical Director of the Missouri Telehealth Network, and Co-Director of the Center for Health Policy at the University of Missouri in Columbia.

DR. JOHN D. WHITED is a research associate with the Health Services Research and Development Service with the Department of Veterans Affairs and an assistant professor of medicine at the Duke University Medical Center in Durham, North Carolina.

TELEDERMATOLOGY
A User's Guide

Edited by

Hon S. Pak

Telemedicine and Advanced Technology Research
Center

Karen E. Edison

University of Missouri

John D. Whited

Duke University Medical Center

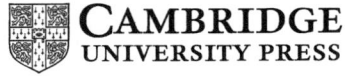

CAMBRIDGE
UNIVERSITY PRESS

CAMBRIDGE UNIVERSITY PRESS
Cambridge, New York, Melbourne, Madrid, Cape Town, Singapore,
São Paulo, Delhi

Cambridge University Press
32 Avenue of the Americas, New York, NY 10013-2473, USA

www.cambridge.org
Information on this title: www.cambridge.org/9780521683357

© Cambridge University Press 2008

First published 2008

Printed in the United States of America

A catalog record for this publication is available from the British Library

Library of Congress Cataloging in Publication Data

Teledermatology : a user's guide / edited by Hon S. Pak, Karen E. Edison,
John D. Whited.
     p. ; cm.
Includes bibliographical references and index.
ISBN 978-0-521-68335-7 (pbk.)
1. Dermatology. 2. Telecommunication in medicine. I. Pak, Hon S., 1964-
II. Edison, Karen E. (Karen Elaine), 1964- III. Whited, John D. (John David), 1962-
[DNLM: 1. Dermatology–organization & administration.
2. Telemedicine–organization & administration. WR 100 T2675 2008]

RL72.T43 2008
616.50068–dc22
2007051327

ISBN 978-0-521-68335-7 paperback

The views expressed in this publication are those of the authors and do not
necessarily represent the position or policy of the United States Department
of Defense or the United States Department of Veterans Affairs.

This book is dedicated to all the individuals who have developed, researched, and supported teledermatology in the past and to those individuals who will, in the future, further advance the field of teledermatology.

Contents

Acknowledgments

Developing this book required the efforts of several experts in the field of teledermatology representing various disciplines. We could not have produced this book without the efforts of our co-authors, Anne E. Burdick, Shasa Hu, Joe Kvedar, Karen Rheuban, Marc Goldyne, Gail Barker, Joseph Tracy, David A. Fleming, Kimberly A. Sackheim, and Daniel Siegel. We offer our sincere thanks for the work put in by these individuals.

We would also like to acknowledge the Teledermatology Special Interest Group of the American Telemedicine Association. Many of the authors of this book are members of this group and share ideas and experiences that contributed to this book.

Finally we would like to thank the publisher, Cambridge University Press. We appreciate their interest, support, and willingness to publish a book on the emerging discipline of teledermatology. We would also like to thank Carlos Aguirre and the team at Cambridge University Press for guiding us through the publication of this book.

List of contributors

Gail Barker
Arizona Telemedicine Program
University of Arizona
Tucson, Arizona, USA

Anne E. Burdick
University of Miami Miller School of Medicine
Miami, Florida, USA

Karen E. Edison
Department of Dermatology and Missouri Telehealth Network
University of Missouri
Columbia, Missouri, USA

David A. Fleming
MU Center for Health Ethics
University of Missouri School of Medicine
Columbia, Missouri, USA

Marc Goldyne
Department of Dermatology
University of California
San Francisco, California, USA

Shasa Hu
Jackson Memorial Hospital Dermatology Program
Miami, Florida, USA

Joseph C. Kvedar
Center for Connected Health
Partners HealthCare System Inc.

Department of Dermatology
Harvard Medical School
Boston, Massachusetts, USA

Hon S. Pak
Telemedicine and Advanced Technology Research Center
Fort Detrick, Maryland, USA

Karen Rheuban
Office of Telemedicine
University of Virginia
Charlottesville, Virginia, USA

Kimberly A. Sackheim
Department of Rehabilitation Medicine
Mount Sinai School of Medicine
New York, New York, USA

Daniel Siegel
Clinical Professor of Dermatology
Director, Procedural Dermatology Fellowship
SUNY Downstate
Brooklyn, New York, USA

Joseph Tracy
Lehigh Valley Hospital and Health Network
Allentown, Pennsylvania, USA

John D. Whited
Center for Health Services Research in Primary Care
Veterans Affairs Medical Center
Division of General Internal Medicine
Duke University Medical Center
Durham, North Carolina, USA

1 Introduction

John D. Whited, Karen E. Edison, and Hon S. Pak

The goal of this book is to provide practical guidance for anyone who is interested in initiating a teledermatology program or expanding their current system. This book was written for a wide audience to include anyone in a private practice, academic center, large multispecialty clinic, state or federal sector.

To build a successful program several features require consideration and each is addressed in turn throughout this book. Specifically, relevant questions include the following:

1. What are your motivating factors? Do you want to increase access for the underserved? Increase your revenue stream? Maximize flexibility in your lifestyle? Or a combination of these factors?
2. What type of technology should you implement – store-and-forward, real-time interactive, or a hybrid model?
3. What are the equipment needs?
4. What communication systems are available for data transmission?
5. Who should be targeted as users (e.g., referring clinicians, patient population, and/or participating teledermatologists)?
6. Is teledermatology a sustainable enterprise and what are the business models that can be followed?
7. Is teledermatology reimbursable and, if so, how?
8. Is image quality good, and what are the training requirements?
9. Is teledermatology a diagnostically viable way of delivering dermatologic healthcare?
10. What legal, regulatory, and confidentiality issues arise?
11. What are the ethical considerations of using the technology?
12. Can teledermatology be integrated into dermatology training programs?

Although this may seem like a daunting list, it should not discourage you from pursuing a teledermatology implementation plan. With proper forethought and planning, the development of a teledermatology program can be tremendously successful. As well as being among the world experts in teledermatology, many of the contributors to this book have developed successful and viable teledermatology programs. The knowledge delivered in this book is based on experience that includes successes, failures, and lessons learned in the course of teledermatology development.

What is teledermatology? Teledermatology, in its simplest terms, is the use of communication information technology to deliver dermatologic care. Typically, technology is used when a conventional "face-to-face" clinic visit cannot be performed – implying that distance or some other barrier prevents this conventional method of healthcare. In these situations the patient and clinician are separated by a geographic barrier, with technology providing the link. This is actually a restricted view of how teledermatology may be used in healthcare delivery but is, nonetheless, a useful way to describe the most common rationale for teledermatology implementation – a patient and a clinician separated from one another by distance. As is described in more detail later, there are two types of unique teledermatology modalities. The first type of modality is real-time interactive patient care, which employs videoconferencing events that use audio-visual communication technologies. The patient and clinician interact with one another in real time and are thereby separated only by space and not time. These are also known as synchronous visits or consults. The second method is called the store-and-forward type. Store-and-forward type interventions use "still" digital images bundled with text-based historical and demographic data. Store-and-forward consults are typically generated and reviewed at different times and are, thus, sometimes referred to as asynchronous consults. Store-and-forward consults separate the patient and clinician in both space and time. Aside from the technology, the major difference between these two types of care delivery is the ability of the patient and clinician to interact with each other when using real-time interactive technology. More recently, a hybrid model has emerged that combines both technologies to leverage the advantages of each teledermatology modality.

Dermatology was an early adopter of telemedicine technology, in large part because of the visual nature of the specialty. Some of the first telemedicine reports in modern medical literature resulted from a telemedicine link between Boston's Logan Airport and the Massachusetts General Hospital in the early 1970s [1]. A telemedicine link was established at a traveler's clinic located within the Logan Airport and was staffed by physicians at the Massachusetts General Hospital. Many of these interventions involved travelers with dermatologic complaints [2]. This particular telemedicine program used videoconferencing (real-time interactive) technology. Telemedicine was relatively quiescent for several years after these reports. A resurgence in interest in the late 1980s and early 1990s coincided with the development of cheaper and more efficient videoconferencing technologies, personal computers, and the Internet. With the digital transformation of healthcare, telemedicine had a natural medium for data transmission. Specifically, digital imaging technology allowed for easy capture, transmission, and review of digitized versions of skin conditions (i.e., digital images) that could be bundled with other digital information. These digital consults could be integrated as part of an electronic medical record or could utilize other existing technology such as web-based interfaces.

Teledermatology is an evolving aspect of healthcare delivery, in part, due to the technology-oriented features inherent to telemedicine. Nonetheless, teledermatology is more rooted in experience and evidence than many other uses of telemedicine technology. In fact, teledermatology has been considered one of the best studied of the telemedicine disciplines [3].

As is described in the literature review chapter (Chapter 4), teledermatology is considered to be a reliable and accurate means of making diagnoses of skin conditions. Successful teledermatology systems have been implemented in the U.S. Department of Veterans Affairs, the U.S. Department of Defense, state-run healthcare programs, academic medical centers, and in private healthcare. Overall, telemedicine has been accepted by practitioners and patients alike in these settings. Reimbursement, specifically federal reimbursement, for teledermatology services (and telemedicine in general) represents the greatest barrier to wider adoption in the United States. Whereas real-time teledermatology interventions can usually bill for services, store-and-forward systems (with some exceptions) cannot. This is an active area of legislation and lobbying, and one that is likely to evolve in the coming years. Interestingly, despite the lack of wide federal reimbursement, utilization of teledermatology appears to be growing. This growth may be a result of an ongoing shortage/maldistribution of dermatologist in the United States. In the conclusion of this book, readers are directed to various web sites and other sources that can provide up-to-date information on this and a myriad other issues that confront teledermatology.

Throughout the book, the following themes and concepts are addressed and integrated into each chapter, as applicable:

1. There is a significant maldistribution of dermatologists. In fact, approximately 40 percent of our population does not have access to dermatological services.
2. Teledermatology utilization is growing in this country and around the world to meet the needs of our patients.
3. Teledermatology primarily improves access to and efficiency of dermatological care delivery. It solves the problem of maldistribution.
4. Teledermatology includes live-interactive, store-and-forward, and hybrid modalities. It may involve primary care provider to dermatologist or patient to dermatologist, depending on the setting.
5. Telecare (direct patient care), teletriage, teleconsultation, and tele-referral services are all possible with teledermatology.
6. Teledermatology is safe, timely, equitable, efficient, effective, and patient centered.
7. Teledermatology technologies are increasingly reliable and affordable.

8. The technology must be adapted based on the particular setting to ensure that it adds value to the organization (education, etc.).
9. Human factors are of greater importance than technology. It is more about people than technology.
10. New models of care delivery, like teledermatology, impact the traditional doctor-patient and doctor-doctor relationship. It allows other care delivery models not previously possible without teledermatology such as remote physician extender supervision and virtual hospital consultation.
11. Teledermatology allows for virtual collaboration among experts for challenging patients nationwide or even worldwide.
12. Teledermatology serves as a new evaluation tool in residency training and enhances overall residency education by allowing objective measurements of the core competencies and access to diverse patient populations, otherwise not possible previously.
13. Teledermatology does not seek to replace dermatologists; it allows greater optimization of our scarce dermatology resources by mitigating distance and/or time barriers to care.
14. The key to successful implementation is in clearly identifying the needs and values of the organization, setting realistic expectations, marketing/education/buy-in, and customizing a solution that minimally disrupts the care delivery process.

REFERENCES

[1] Murphy RLH, Bird KT. Telediagnosis: A new community health resource. Observations on the feasibility of telediagnosis based on 1000 patient transactions. *Am J Public Health* 1974;64:113–19.
[2] Murphy RLH, Fitzpatrick TB, Haynes HA, Bird KT, Sheridan TB. Accuracy of dermatologic diagnosis by television. *Arch Dermatol* 1972;105:833–5.
[3] *Telemedicine for the Medicare Population*. Summary, Evidence Report/Technology Assessment: Number 24. AHRQ Publication Number 01-E011, February 2001. Agency for Healthcare Research and Quality, Rockville, MD. http://www.ahrq.gov/clinic/epcsums/telemedsum.htm. Last accessed on August 16, 2007.

2 Teledermatology modalities

Hon S. Pak, Karen E. Edison, and John D. Whited

There are three major teledermatology modalities. Live-interactive and store-and-forward are the two most common modalities with the hybrid model that includes elements of both live-interactive and store-and-forward technologies emerging as the third new modality. Each modality has its advantages and disadvantages and selection is based on the needs of the organization, the dermatology resources available, the teledermatology visit and/or consult volume, existing communication infrastructure, and the objectives of the program.

Live-interactive teledermatology

Live-interactive teledermatology takes advantage of videoconferencing as its core technology. Participants are separated by distance, but interact in real time. Thus, live-interactive patient visits are also known as synchronous visits or consults. By convention, the site where the patient is located is referred to as the *originating site* and the site where the consultant is located is referred to as the *distant site*. A high-resolution camera or monitor is required at the originating site. Videoconferencing systems work optimally when a connection speed of 384 kbps or higher is used. Slower connection speeds may necessitate that the individual presenting the patient perform either a still-image capture or a freeze-frame to render a diagnostic image. For most diagnostic images, a minimum resolution of 800×600 pixels (480,000) is required.

Live-interactive interactions are initiated similar to in-person dermatological care. Patients may make their own teledermatology appointments or a referring provider may request the visit. A live-interactive appointment is scheduled in a manner similar to that of conventional clinic-based visits. A telepresenter is present at the originating site to facilitate the consultation. This could be the referring clinician, but it is often a nurse or other health professional. The telepresenter initiates the videoconferencing telemedicine (VTC) visit and is available to assist in obtaining any information, including imaging, that is necessary to make a diagnosis and management plan.

Live-interactive visits can be used for telereferral, teleconsultation, teletriage, and direct telecare. The referring provider can assume responsibility for patient management based on recommendations provided by the consulting dermatologist or the dermatologist can be responsible for the patient's care.

A major advantage of live-interactive technology is the ability of the dermatologist and patient to interact with one another. The dermatologist can obtain a history, ask directed questions, and view all parts of the skin surface. Other than the inability to palpate the skin condition which is not possible with current technology, the visit otherwise closely mimics conventional care. The training requirements for using the videoconferencing equipment are moderate. Additionally, there is the potential for the referring clinician to derive an educational benefit from the consult, particularly if he or she participates in the teledermatology consult.

One disadvantage of live-interactive teledermatology, compared with store-and-forward care, is that dermatologists are fixed to a schedule much like the structure of a conventional clinic. The originating and distant sites must interact in real time which requires agreement on a scheduled time. Also, the bandwidth requirements necessary to achieve adequate resolution in a videoconferencing session can be costly.

Live-interactive teledermatology is best utilized when communication with the patient and patient education are important elements of the patient-physician interaction. Live-interactive teledermatology can also provide more intensive and interactive training for the referring clinician if he or she participates in the consultation.

Store-and-forward teledermatology

Store-and-forward teledermatology utilizes a set of digital "still" images bundled with what is typically a standardized set of historical and demographic information. A store-and-forward teledermatology consult is analogous to an email system that includes text-based historical information with digital images as attachments. As the name implies, the teledermatology consult is generated and reviewed at different times and therefore represents an asynchronous consult system. The teledermatology consult is generated at the referring site and is forwarded to the site of dermatology consultation. Generally, this is generated by a healthcare professional (e.g., nurse) who has received training in the imaging and consult generation protocol, but can be performed by non-clinicians (e.g., technicians) if adequately trained. After receiving the teledermatology consultation, the dermatologist then generates a report that is sent back to the referring site. This would include a diagnosis, or presumptive diagnosis, and a management plan that is implemented by the referring clinician.

Store-and-forward teledermatology can be used in teleconsultation, telereferral, telecare, or teletriage care delivery mode. Most commonly store-and-forward teledermatology is used in teleconsultation.

If a referring provider has integrated the teledermatology consult system into his/her practice, store-and-forward teledermatology can be an on-demand service in a manner similar to laboratory tests and radiological tests. Alternatively, teledermatology can be scheduled as a periodic service (e.g., twice a month), particularly if the setting would be expected to generate low volume of consults.

An advantage of store-and-forward teledermatology is that it is more scalable for high volume given its ability to optimize the capacity of dermatologists. When teledermatology referrals are integrated into the referring provider's clinic, patients benefit from the convenience of not having to travel to another clinic at another site. Because of the asynchronous nature of the consult process, dermatologists can review cases and complete consults at times and locations that are most convenient. Dedicated time that must coincide with the referral site is not necessary.

One of the disadvantages of store-and-forward teledermatology is that adequate training is required to ensure that imaging is done correctly and imaging protocols are followed properly. Quality assurance is an important element of this type of consult generation. Also, there is no direct contact between the dermatologist and the patient; consequently, counseling and education interventions are hindered if not prevented in this format. Referring provider contact education is indirect with store-and-forward teledermatology.

Store-and-forward teledermatology is best used when bandwidth requirements are unavailable or prohibitively costly. When dermatologist time cannot be dedicated to a mutually agreeable time between the referring site and the consulting site, store-and-forward teledermatology is advantageous. Store-and-forward teledermatology works well for high-volume settings. This is because store-and-forward consults generally require less time to perform than live-interactive consults.

Hybrid model

The hybrid model merges elements of live-interactive and store-and-forward teledermatology and, therefore, benefits from the advantages and strengths of both models. With a hybrid model the videoconferencing equipment does not require a high-resolution imaging device as this feature is used primarily for patient-physician interaction. High-resolution digital still images of the affected area are presented to the dermatologist during the consultation. This eliminates the need for expert video camera operation at the originating site. Although high-end videoconferencing systems are commonly used in hybrid teledermatology, a webcam or videophone could be used as the interactive technology.

Hybrid consults are initiated by the referring provider or the patient. The patient returns for a later teledermatology appointment. The nurse (telepresenter) obtains the digital still images and history a few minutes prior to the scheduled live-interactive appointment time. The still images can be either forwarded to the dermatologist before the scheduled appointment time or presented during the live-interactive examination. The recommendations can be provided to the referring provider who can then manage the patient or the teledermatologist can take primary responsibility and prescribe the course of treatment.

The hybrid model can be used for telecare, telereferral, teletriage, and teleconsultation. Depending on the arrangement, the referring provider or the consulting dermatologist can be responsible for managing the patient. Scheduling for the hybrid model occurs in the same manner as stand-alone live-interactive teledermatology.

An advantage of the hybrid model is that it combines some features of both types of consult modalities. Physician-patient interaction is maintained. High-quality digital still images are available, thus averting time lost in obtaining high-quality video images, such as of a restless child. This system also avoids the need for large bandwidth connections since the still images can be forwarded over low bandwidth lines – high-quality video images are not necessary. This reduces the cost of hybrid systems over live-interactive only systems. Hybrid models also require synchronization of referring site and consulting site scheduling. A fixed schedule analogous to conventional clinic scheduling is required.

Hybrid models are useful when a combination of store-and-forward and live-interactive elements are desired. The physician-patient interaction is maintained, but the quality of visual information obtained does not require high bandwidth connections or expert video camera performance. The high-resolution images of the involved area are forwarded as still images.

3 Telemedicine implementation and reimbursement surveys

Anne E. Burdick and Shasa Hu

Association of Telehealth Service Providers (ATSP) Surveys

The ATSP published annual reports from 1997 to 2001 that included information on U.S. teledermatology services [1]. The 2001 report was based on a questionnaire sent to 206 telemedicine programs. The report provided information on the 82 telemedicine programs that responded and included the clinical specialties provided. The ATSP report did not include reimbursement information.

2002 AMD Telemedicine/American Telemedicine Association (ATA) Reimbursement Survey

In 2002, AMD Telemedicine and the ATA conducted a survey of telemedicine reimbursement [2]. The initial survey was sent to approximately 2,000 ATA members. Despite a poor response rate, ATA and AMD Telemedicine identified 141 active U.S. telemedicine programs with 72 of the 141 programs that billed for telemedicine services. These 72 programs were then surveyed by telephone. The survey revealed that 38 of the 72 programs (53%) were reimbursed for telemedicine services by private payers and that 150 private payers reimbursed for telemedicine in 24 states. Blue Cross/Blue Shield reimbursed in 13 states whereas Medicaid reimbursed in only 18 states. Four states had legislations mandating private payer reimbursement of telemedicine services: California SB 1665 (1996), Kentucky HB 177 (2000), Louisiana SB 773 (1995), and Texas HB 2033 (1997). Detailed survey results were posted on the "Private Payer Reimbursement Information Directory" web site (http://www.amdtelemedicine.com/private_payer/index.cfm), which is regularly updated with private payers and states in which Medicaid reimburses for telemedicine. As of June 2005, Blue Cross/Blue Shield reimbursed for telemedicine services in 21 states. The Oklahoma state legislation mandated private payers to reimburse for telemedicine services (Oklahoma SB 48, 1997).

The 2002 AMD/ATA survey identified strategies that telemedicine programs used to obtain private payer reimbursement. Some programs sent letters to private payers stating that the programs intended to provide telemedicine services and that in the future, bills would be submitted for these services. Although the programs asked for questions and/or comments from the insurance companies, none responded. Few telemedicine providers use modifiers and/or specialized CPT codes for tracking services. Most do not and submit claims in the usual and customary manner. Therefore, data collection for this survey was difficult to obtain. In addition, reimbursement was not categorized by the type of telemedicine (store-and-forward [SF] vs live-interactive [LI]) or clinical specialties. Some programs did not share their contractual arrangements.

ATA Teledermatology Special Interest Group Reimbursement Survey

Little information existed on teledermatology reimbursement prior to 2000. In December 2000, the Telemedicine Research Center (Portland, OR) sent a teledermatology survey to the six most active teledermatology networks and received responses from four programs: University of California-Davis, University of Missouri, University of Arizona, and Mountaineer Doctor Television at West Virginia University [3]. The survey questions focused on activity and structure of teledermatology services. Although there were no survey questions on reimbursement, all four networks reported receiving reimbursement for consultations. University of California-Davis was reimbursed by the state's Medicaid system, Medi-Cal, as mandated by the California Telemedicine Development Act of 1996, and also by Blue Cross of California.

One other teledermatology reimbursement survey was conducted in January 2003 which was sent by email by the Association of Dermatology Administrators to all academic dermatology programs, but the response rate was low.

In June 2003, the ATA Teledermatology Special Interest Group attempted to determine the extent of teledermatology activity and reimbursement for U.S. teledermatology services [4]. Five hundred questionnaires were emailed to all ATA members, U.S. dermatology program administrators, and various web databases (Table 3-1). The survey questions were:

1. Are you doing teledermatology?
2. If yes, is LI and/or SF teledermatology offered?
3. How many consults did you perform in 2002?
4. Are you being reimbursed? If yes, are you being reimbursed by private payer, Medicaid, Medicare, or self-pay?

Over the next 3 months, a database of teledermatology programs was created based on the responses that included information from the Association

Table 3-1: Sources for ATA Teledermatology Special Interest Group Survey distribution list

⟹ ATA members: programs and individuals
⟹ ATA Teledermatology Special Interest Group participants at the 2003 annual meeting
⟹ AMD Telemedicine/ATA Private Payer Survey 2002, Debra VanderWerf
⟹ ATSP 2001 Survey
⟹ TIE
⟹ U.S. Dermatology Residency Programs
⟹ Association of Dermatology Administrators

of Dermatology Administrators January 2003 survey, the AMD Telemedicine/ATA private payer 2002 survey, the 2001 ATSP survey and the Telemedicine Information Exchange (TIE) web site database. The last two surveys provided a list of potential programs active in teledermatology. Since the ATSP survey was conducted in 2001 and the TIE web site was created several years prior, a telephone call was made to the telemedicine program coordinators of these programs to confirm the accuracy of the information posted. Those programs that responded to the initial survey and/or to follow-up phone calls were categorized as either "Active" or "Not Active" in teledermatology based on whether they were offering teledermatology at the time. This survey's response rate was approximately 24%.

Of 106 programs in the database on 2002 teledermatology activity, 62 were active in teledermatology, 5 were starting teledermatology, and 4 had previously offered teledermatology. At least 36 states had a teledermatology program (Figure 3-1). A majority of the programs was affiliated with an academic center or the military/Veterans Affairs (VA) system. Seven programs had contracts with the Department of Correction (DOC). Examples of academic teledermatology programs with resident participation included University of Kansas, at which LI teledermatology consultations were performed to serve rural patients. At programs such as the University of Miami, SF teledermatology was utilized at an HIV/AIDS clinic. A few programs served populations with special needs: East Carolina University conducted LI teledermatology to treat patients from the State Mental Health Hospital, Home for the Mentally Retarded, and School for the Deaf. Two programs specialized in LI pediatric teledermatology: Children's Hospital and Regional Medical Center at Washington and Children's Hospital in Los Angeles.

The highest volumes of consults (average of 577 per year) were seen in military/VA-affiliated programs. The second highest number of consults were at programs serving a prison population (average of 252 per year) (Figure 3-2 and Table 3-2). Figure 3-2 illustrates the mean consult volume in

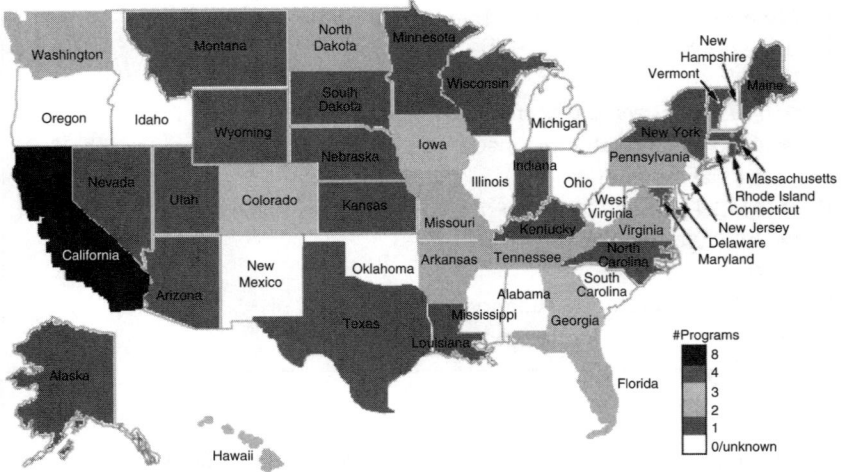

Figure 3-1 States with active teledermatology programs

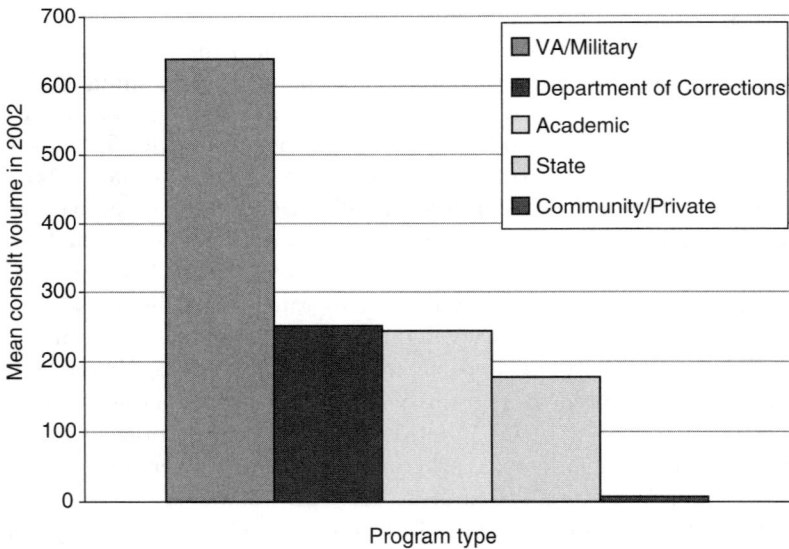

Figure 3-2 Teledermatology consult volume

2002 by program types. Interestingly, the survey results indicated that California and Texas had the most number of programs, eight and four, respectively, which may be related to the fact that these two states had legislation that mandated private payer reimbursement for telemedicine services (Figure 3-1).

Table 3-2: Teledermatology consult volume

Program affiliation	Range of consults in 2002	Mean consult volume in 2002
Military/VA	50 to 1,500	639
State	5 to 400	178
Department of Correction	85 to 400	252
Academic programs	<10 to 500–700	245
Community/Private	2 to 15	7

LI technology was more commonly used for teledermatology consults compared to SF technology. Of the programs that responded, 34 programs performed LI teledermatology services (14 of which were based in academic dermatology programs), 17 programs offered SF services (10 of which were military/VA based), and 7 programs had both LI and SF teledermatology. Four programs had terminated teledermatology services and the reasons included "not enough interest" and "dermatologist left the practice."

More than half of the active programs (49 of 62) responded to the survey questions on reimbursement status and mode of teledermatology services. Thirty-nine of forty-nine programs (78%) received reimbursement, some from more than one payer. Private payers and Medicare were the most frequent reimbursement sources followed by federal funding and contracts with DOC. Eighteen programs were reimbursed by private payers, sixteen programs by Medicaid, twelve programs by Medicare, eight programs by patient self-pay, and twenty-seven programs by other sources such as federal grants, DOC, or military contracts.

Information on reimbursement was then collated with the type of teledermatology system (Figures 3-3 and 3-4). Eighteen states reimbursed LI teledermatology consults by Medicaid. Medicare reimbursed LI teleconsultations with certain restrictions. LI consults were reimbursed more often than SF consults. Most LI-only programs, 21 of 24 programs (88%), received reimbursement, mainly from Medicare and private payers including Blue Cross Medicaid (Medi-Cal) and Blue Cross Healthy Families in California and Blue Cross/Blue Shield in Kansas and North Dakota. In comparison, 11 of 17 SF-only programs (65%) were reimbursed, mostly from federal grants, DOC, or military/VA contracts.

The ATA SIG survey was conducted over a 3-month period from June through September 2003 and provided a "snapshot" of teledermatology activity and reimbursement. Although the response rate was limited, the list of surveyees was comprehensive as it incorporated databases from multiple previous telemedicine surveys and major telemedicine and dermatology organizations. While most of the large active telemedicine programs

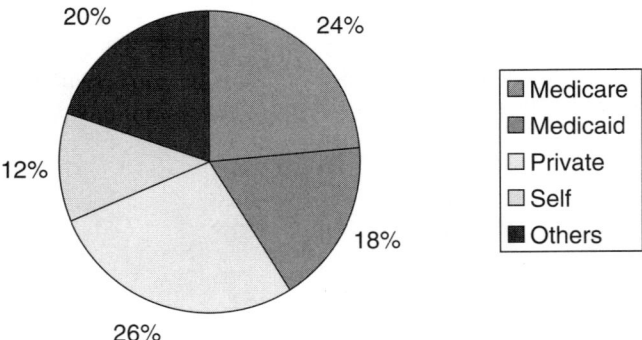

Figure 3-3 Reimbursement sources for live-interactive teledermatology consults in 2003
Note: Others – Department of Correction contracts, Department of Defense contracts, military funds, Veteran Administration funds, Office for the Advancement of Telehealth (OAT) grants, and other state or federal government grants.

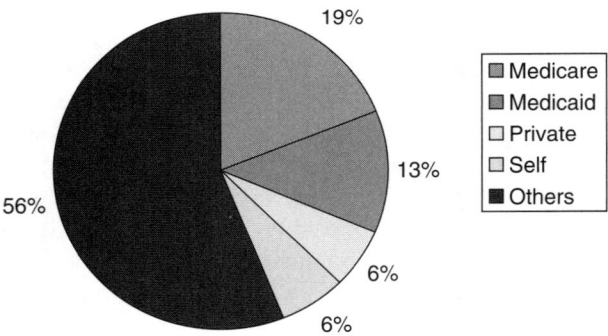

Figure 3-4 Reimbursement sources for Store-forward teledermatology consults in 2003
Note: Others – Department of Correction contracts, Department of Defense contracts, military funds, Veteran Administration funds, Office for the Advancement of Telehealth (OAT) grants, and other state or federal government grants.

responded fully to the survey, it is likely that some practitioners who provided teledermatology consultations may not have been emailed with the questionnaire. As with the AMD/ATA survey, some responders did not disclose their reimbursement sources.

REFERENCES

[1] Association of Telehealth Service Providers. 2001 ATSP Report on U.S. Telemedicine Activity. Portland, OR, 2001.

[2] Vanderwerf D. 2002 Survey of private payer reimbursement for telemedicine. American Telemedicine Association and AMD Telemedicine. http://www. amdtelemedicine.com/private_payer/index.cfm. Last accessed on June 8, 2005.

[3] Grigsby B, Brown NA. A survey of teledermatology in the USA. In R Wootton, AMM Oakley (eds), *Teledermatology*. London: Royal Society of Medicine Press, 2002, pp. 59–69.

[4] Burdick AE, Hu S. Current status of US teledermatology activities and reimbursement survey. Presented at 2004 Ninth Annual Meeting and Exposition of the American Telemedicine Association. Tampa, FL. http://www.atmeda.org/ news/2004_presentations/m1c4.burdick.ppt. Last accessed on September 1, 2007.

4 Review of literature

John D. Whited

Introduction

"What evidence do you have that teledermatology is effective?" is a question that may be posed by an administrator when asked to support a teledermatology program. This chapter provides some answers to that likely query by reviewing the current status of teledermatology research. Teledermatology is one of the best-studied fields of telemedicine. Research has been conducted on diagnostic reliability and accuracy, management outcomes, clinical outcomes, satisfaction assessments, and economic analyses. Using these research categories, this chapter concisely summarizes the status of teledermatology research. Although this summary is not a critique of research methodology, only those studies that are of sufficient quality to arrive at reasonable conclusions are included. These conclusions will be reported in a summary statement at the end of each section. Despite the relatively large number of studies that address teledermatology, the body of teledermatology research is far from complete. Therefore, this chapter concludes with a description of directions for future research.

For those readers less familiar with research terminology, the following is a description of the terms that will be used throughout this chapter. For those interested, further information can be found in textbooks by Sackett et al. and Fletcher et al. and in a previously published review [1–3].

When research is conducted on a new diagnostic modality (teledermatology) compared to a conventional modality (clinic-based examination), two diagnostic features are typically described, namely *diagnostic reliability* and *diagnostic accuracy*. Reliability simply refers to agreement. If two examiners independently reach the same diagnosis they are in agreement and are displaying diagnostic reliability. Even if both examiners are providing an incorrect diagnosis (see accuracy below) their diagnoses are nonetheless reliable because they have provided the same diagnosis. In addition to agreement, other synonyms for reliability are repeatability, reproducibility, concordance, and precision. *Interobserver reliability* refers to reliability measured between two or more different examiners and *intraobserver reliability* refers to reliability measured between one examiner with his or her self over serial reviews. *Accuracy* describes whether the diagnosis offered is correct or incorrect. Diagnostic accuracy is evaluated by comparing the diagnosis with a *gold standard test*. The gold standard test is considered to be the best available test for classifying the presence or absence of disease. An example of a gold standard test in dermatology is histopathological review of biopsied tissue to determine the presence or absence of a malignant skin condition.

The accuracy of a diagnostic test is reported in terms of its *sensitivity* and *specificity*. Sensitivity answers the question, among patients who truly have the disease, what proportion will have a positive diagnostic test result? A highly sensitive test will yield a positive test result in nearly every patient who has the disease. That is a desirable feature if the consequences of missing the disease of interest have potentially grave clinical consequences. However, a highly sensitive test may classify nearly everyone as having the disease, even if they do not have the disease. That is where the concept of specificity becomes important. Specificity answers the question, among patients who truly do *not* have the disease, how many will have a negative test result? A highly specific test will yield a negative test result in nearly every patient who does not have the disease. Ideally, a test should be both highly sensitive and specific so that it correctly identifies those patients who have the disease of interest and correctly identifies those who do not have the disease of interest. In reality, there are often trade-offs between sensitivity and specificity, so that as a test's sensitivity increases it often does so at the expense of specificity, and vice versa.

When reporting economic analyses, the *economic perspective* of that study should be described. The economic perspective considers the economic impact from a specific point of view. Examples of economic perspectives include the *societal perspective* (all the costs borne by society at large) and a subset of societal costs such as those borne by a particular healthcare system. A *cost analysis* is an accounting of the cost, irrespective of effectiveness or benefit, for an intervention. A *cost-effectiveness* analysis compares the incremental cost and incremental effectiveness of two or more interventions. The units of effectiveness are nonmonetary and generally reflect some clinical outcome (e.g., days of hospitalization avoided). Cost-effectiveness analyses are the most common method of reporting economic analyses. A *cost-benefit* analysis reports all costs and outcomes analysis in monetary terms. This requires, of course, that the outcome be reportable with a monetary value. A *cost-minimization* analysis compares the incurred costs of two or more interventions that achieve, or are expected to achieve, the same outcome (i.e., there is no expected advantage in effectiveness between options).

Diagnostic reliability

Store and forward

INTEROBSERVER RELIABILITY

Interobserver reliability can be measured between a clinic-based dermatologist and another clinic-based dermatologist, between a clinic-based
dermatologist and a teledermatologist, and between a teledermatologist and
another teledermatologist. Interobserver reliability found between teledermatologists and clinic-based dermatologists, reported as simple agreement, has ranged from 41% to 95% [4–16] (Table 4-1). As might be expected,
agreement increases when alternative or differential diagnoses are considered, as opposed to rating agreement based solely on the single most likely
diagnosis.

One of these studies employed multiple examinations of the same
patient sample to place interobserver reliability assessments in the context of
a "baseline" level of agreement found among different clinic-based dermatologists [8]. The level of agreement found between different clinic-based

Table 4-1: Interobserver reliability between clinic-based
dermatologists and teledermatologists using store-and-forward
technology – point estimate data reported as simple agreement

Reference	Complete agreement (%)	Partial agreement (%)
Kvedar [4]	61–64	67–70
Zelickson [5]	88	NA
Lyon [6]	89	NA
High [7]	64–77	81–89
Whited [8]	41–55	79–95
Taylor [9]	44–51	57–61
Lim [10]	73–85	83–89
Eminovic [11]	41	51
Du Moulin [12]	54	63
Mahendran [13]	44–48	64–65
Oakley [14]	53	64
Tucker [15]	56	68
Bowns [16]	55	NA

Note: Complete agreement – considers the single most likely diagnosis; partial
agreement – considers both the single most likely diagnosis and differential diagnoses
or comparable diagnoses; NA, not available.

dermatologists was 54% (95% confidence interval, 46–61%) when only the single most likely diagnosis was considered and was 92% (95% confidence interval, 88–96%) when differential diagnoses were considered. This compared favorably to agreement found between clinic-based dermatologists and teledermatologists. Agreement between these two types of examiners ranged from 41% to 55% (95% confidence interval range, 34–63%) based on the single most likely diagnosis and from 83% to 95% (95% confidence interval range, 78–98%) when differential diagnoses were considered. Different teledermatologists performing teledermatology consultations also demonstrated comparable reliability to that found between the other two groups. Teledermatologists agreed with one another at a rate ranging from 49% to 55% (95% confidence interval range, 41–63%) for agreement on the single most likely diagnosis and from 84% to 92% (95% confidence interval range, 79–96%) when differential diagnoses were included in the analysis.

The kappa statistic is used when correcting for agreement expected by chance. Although somewhat arbitrary, a kappa of 0.61 or higher is considered a substantially higher level of agreement than would be expected by chance alone and is generally accepted as a benchmark of high reliability [17]. The kappa statistic can be used only when diagnoses can be placed into discrete categories. Four studies have analyzed reliability using the kappa statistic – one study categorized the data based on whether the examiners considered a lesion to represent a benign or malignant condition and the others used lesion categories that included benign and malignant presentations [8, 18–20] (Table 4-2). All studies reported kappa statistics that would be considered substantially higher than that expected by chance.

INTRAOBSERVER RELIABILITY
Table 4-3 summarizes studies of intraobserver agreement measured between the same examiner reviewing a patient in a clinic setting vs their review of that patient's teledermatology consultation. Although intraobserver agreement levels are typically higher than interobserver agreement values, the range of agreement was similar for that found for interobserver agreement.

Real-time interactive

INTEROBSERVER RELIABILITY
Interobserver agreement between teledermatologists and clinic-based dermatologists when using real-time interactive technology has ranged from 54% to 99%, reported as simple proportion agreement [22–28] (Table 4-4). The range of agreement for real-time interactive technology (54–99%) is similar to that found for store-and-forward techniques (41–95%).

One of these studies [22] also measured the level interobserver agreement found between two clinic-based examiners to provide a context for the

Table 4-2: Diagnostic reliability measures using the kappa statistic

Reference	Lesion category	Agreement category	Examiner pairings	Kappa	95% CI ranges
Whited [8]	Malignancy	Complete	Clinic based vs clinic based	0.68	0.52–0.83
Whited [8]	Malignancy	Complete	Teledermatologist vs teledermatologist	0.68	0.59–0.77
Whited [8]	Malignancy	Partial	Clinic based vs clinic based	0.77	0.62–0.92
Whited [8]	Malignancy	Partial	Teledermatologist vs teledermatologist	0.63	0.55–0.72
Krupinski [18]	Various lesion types	Partial	Clinic based vs teledermatologist	0.80–0.82	NA
Baba [19]	Various lesion types	Complete	Teledermatologist vs teledermatologist	0.71	0.60–0.82
Moreno-Ramirez [20]	Various lesion types	Complete	Teledermatologist vs teledermatologist	0.91	0.87–0.96
Moreno-Ramirez [20]	Various lesion types	Complete	Clinic based vs teledermatologist	0.90	0.90–1.0

Note: Complete agreement – considers the single most likely diagnosis; partial agreement – considers both the single most likely diagnosis and differential diagnoses; NA, not available.

Table 4-3: Intraobserver diagnostic reliability between clinic-based evaluations and store-and-forward teledermatology evaluations – point estimate data reported as simple agreement

Reference	Complete agreement (%)	Partial agreement (%)
Taylor [9]	31–64	50–70
Lim [10]	88	95
Pak [21]	70	91
Krupinski [18]	NA	76–90

Note: Complete agreement – considers the single most likely diagnosis; partial agreement – considers both the single most likely diagnosis and differential diagnoses; NA, not available.

Table 4-4: Interobserver diagnostic reliability between clinic-based dermatologists and teledermatologists using real-time interactive technology – point estimate data reported as simple agreement

Reference	Complete agreement (%)	Partial agreement (%)
Lesher [22]	78	99
Gilmour [23]	54	80
Lowitt [24]	80	NA
Loane [25]	60	76
Phillips [26]	77	NA
Phillips [27]	59	NA
Nordal [28]	72	86

Note: Complete agreement – considers the single most likely diagnosis; partial agreement – considers both the single most likely diagnosis and differential diagnoses; NA, not available.

level of intermodality reliability. Like the store-and-forward study [8], a comparable level of agreement was found between examiner pairings as evidenced by the overlapping confidence intervals. Clinic-based examiners agreed with one another in 94% (95% confidence interval, 87–100%) of the cases (complete agreement) and 100% of the cases (partial agreement). The clinic-based examiner and teledermatologist pairing yielded an agreement rate of 78% (95% confidence interval, 68–88%) complete agreement and 99% (95% confidence interval, 97–100%) partial agreement.

Table 4-5: Intraobserver diagnostic reliability between clinic-based dermatologists and teledermatologists – point estimate data reported as simple agreement

Reference	Complete agreement (%)	Partial agreement (%)
Gilmour [23]	59	76
Loane [25]	71	87

Note: Complete agreement – considers the single most likely diagnosis; partial agreement – considers both the single most likely diagnosis and differential diagnoses.

INTRAOBSERVER RELIABILITY

Two studies that have reported intraobserver agreement among clinic-based examiners and teledermatologists using real-time interactive technology (Table 4-5). The range of intraobserver agreement was similar to that found for interobserver agreement, as was seen for store-and-forward techniques.

Summary of diagnostic reliability research

The largest and strongest body of research exists regarding the diagnostic reliability of teledermatology. The evidence shows that teledermatology consultations, whether using store-and-forward or real-time interactive techniques, result in highly reliable diagnoses that compare favorably with conventional clinic-based care. This conclusion is based on the repeatability of high simple proportion agreement found in multiple research studies, studies that made simultaneous assessments of "baseline" reliability found among different clinic-based examiners, and reports that used chance-corrected measures of agreement. Additional studies that assess the level of agreement found among different clinic-based examiners while simultaneously evaluating agreement between clinic-based dermatologist and teledermatologist pairings would be the most beneficial study design for future reliability assessments.

Management outcomes

Store and forward

Three studies have assessed the reliability of biopsy recommendations between a teledermatologist and an in-person dermatologist (Table 4-6). The results varied but overall, a moderately good to perfect level of agreement was observed for biopsy recommendations.

Table 4-6: Interobserver agreement between clinic-based examiners and teledermatologists for biopsy recommendations

Reference	Simple agreement (%)	Kappa	95% CI range for kappa
Pak [29]	76	0.47	0.39–0.56
Shapiro [30]	100	1.0	0.72–1.0
Whited [31]	90–100	NA	NA

Note: NA, not available.

One study compared three different categories of management recommendations between different clinic-based examiners, clinic-based examiners and teledermatologists, and different teledermatologists examiners [8]. For medical therapy recommendations, all three groups showed comparable reliability. Clinic-based therapy recommendations showed less reliability than medical therapy recommendations, but were still largely reliable. Diagnostic testing recommendations, which included biopsy decisions, were not reliable. Another study found that the management plan of the clinic-based dermatologist agreed with the teledermatologist in 90% of the cases [6]. Among 43% (70/163) of patients referred for minor operations (including biopsies) after a teledermatology consult, 54 of those (77%) were considered appropriately referred when compared to the results of the conventional clinic-based visit [13]. The remaining 16 (23%) were considered inappropriately referred based on (a) referral for the wrong procedure, (b) a procedure was not required, or (c) a more complex intervention was required.

Real-time interactive

One study that assessed the reliability of biopsy recommendations between a teledermatologist and an in-person dermatologist found an agreement rate of 86% which corresponded to a kappa value of 0.47 (95% confidence interval, 0.24–0.71) [27]. One other study that assessed agreement by categories of treatment plans between a teledermatologist and a clinic-based dermatologist found agreement in 72% of cases [23]. In yet another study, the management plan was rated to be the same or similar in 64% of cases [32]. Of note, in 19% of the cases the teledermatologist could not arrive at a management plan.

Summary of management outcomes research

High simple agreement has been found for biopsy decisions made by teledermatologists and clinic-based dermatologists when using both store-and-forward and real-time interactive techniques. Using kappa statistics, the strength of agreement has ranged from moderate to perfect. Management reliability is arguably of secondary importance to diagnostic reliability, due to variation in treatment preferences found among dermatologists. Management of skin conditions is an intermediary step linking a diagnosis with a clinical outcome. A management strategy, in and of itself, does not necessarily predict a clinical outcome.

Diagnostic accuracy

Diagnostic accuracy assessments for dermatologic disease are somewhat problematic. Histopathologic review of biopsied tissue can function as a gold standard; however, it is primarily a gold standard for determining the presence or absence of malignancy. Histopathologic review cannot be universally used to make a definitive diagnosis of all skin lesions. Even when it is used for suspected benign conditions, the histopathology often only supports a particular diagnosis rather than providing definitive proof of its existence. Furthermore, a skin condition must be observed before it can be biopsied – lesions that are missed during the examination cannot be subjected to a gold standard test. Of course, the entirety of the skin surface cannot be biopsied so lesions that are missed contribute to a false negative rate. Therefore, diagnostic accuracy assessments of dermatologic conditions are somewhat constrained. In some cases, authors have used clinic-based dermatologists' findings as a pragmatic gold standard. While this is a potentially viable technique when a gold standard test does not exist, those studies are reported as diagnostic reliability data as detailed above.

Store and forward

Studies that report diagnostic accuracy appear in Table 4-7. Four studies that analyzed data among a subset of patients that underwent a biopsy and/or had other reference standard tests (e.g., KOH preparation) found comparable diagnostic accuracy between clinic-based examiners and tele-dermatologists [8, 14, 18, 20]. Less conclusive studies correlated histo-pathologic review with traditional photographs and referral letters [33] and analyzed a very small sample size [31].

Real-time interactive

To date, no studies have been published that make accuracy assessments of diagnoses provided through real-time interactive consult methods other than those that have used the pragmatic reference standard of a clinic-based dermatologists' diagnoses. Those studies appear in the diagnostic reliability section.

Table 4-7: Diagnostic accuracy rates by consult modality

Reference	Modality	Complete accuracy rate	95% CI ranges	Partial accuracy rate	95% CI ranges
Whited [8]	Clinic based	0.59–0.71	0.48–0.81	0.85	0.77–0.93
	Teledermatology	0.53–0.63	0.42–0.74	0.68–0.85	0.58–0.93
Krupinski [18]	Clinic based	NA	NA	0.80–0.97[a]	NA
	Teledermatology	NA	NA	0.73–0.78[a]	NA
Harrison [33]	Clinic based	NA	NA	NA	NA
	Teledermatology	0.71	NA	NA	NA
Whited [31]	Clinic based	0.70–0.77	NA	0.80–0.92	NA
	Teledermatology	0.31–0.85	NA	0.85	NA
Moreno-Ramirez [20]	Teledermatology	0.79	NA	NA	NA
Oakley [14]	Clinic based	0.72	0.53–0.87	NA	NA
	Teledermatology	0.71	0.56–0.83	NA	NA

Notes: Complete accuracy – accuracy based on the single most likely diagnosis; partial accuracy – accuracy based on single most likely and differential diagnoses; NA, not available.
[a]No statistical difference by chi-square testing.

Summary of diagnostic accuracy research

Existing evidence, albeit limited in quantity, indicates that store-and-forward teledermatology results in comparable diagnostic accuracy when compared to conventional clinic-based care. This is based on four studies that found comparable diagnostic accuracy between teledermatologists and clinic-based examiners using histopathologic review of biopsied tissue or other reference standard tests to make these assessments [8, 14, 18, 20]. Other less rigorous studies found similar point estimate accuracy rates. No information has been published on the diagnostic accuracy of real-time interactive teledermatology using reference standard tests.

Clinical outcomes

Most published studies to date have evaluated only intermediate clinical outcomes such as consults avoided, time to intervention, and consult-related logistical issues including consult time requirements. With one notable exception, no large published studies have evaluated definitive clinical endpoints such as clinical course, used disease-specific instruments to rate clinical status, or measured quality of life. One large randomized trial did compare the clinical course of store-and-forward teledermatology compared to usual care [34].

Store and forward

One small study made a retrospective assessment of the clinical course of 50 patients who were managed with clinic visits and 50 patients who were managed with store-and-forward teledermatology [35]. Data for rating the clinical course was only available for seven patients – three teledermatology patients and four usual care patients. All three of the teledermatology patients were rated as "improved" and three of the four usual care patients were rate as "improved" with one rated as "unchanged."

A randomized trial made a clinical course assessment between base-line and 4 months for patients undergoing teledermatology consultations compared to a conventional referral process [34]. There was no evidence to suggest a difference in the proportion of clinical course ratings between the two groups. Clinical course was rated on a three-point scale (Table 4-8).

Nine studies have evaluated the proportion of store-and-forward teledermatology consults that did avoid, or would have avoided, a clinic visit to a dermatologist (Table 4-9). The proportion of dermatology clinic visits avoided has ranged from 13% to 53%. The referral setting likely influences rates of clinic visit avoidance. Geographic barriers and the ability or desire of nondermatologists to perform diagnostic or therapeutic interventions (e.g., biopsies) are factors that could affect clinic visit rates in a particular teledermatology consult system. One of these studies [36] used traditional

Table 4-8: Results of the Pak et al. study that rated clinical outcomes

Consult modality	Clinical course rating (%)		
	Improved	No change	Worse
Usual care	65.3	32.2	2.5
Teledermatology	63.6	32.7	3.7

Table 4-9: Dermatology clinic visits avoided with store-and-forward teledermatology

Reference	Dermatology clinic visits avoided (%)
Loane [36]	31 (30/96)
Taylor [9]	31 (118/376)
White [37]	25 (10/40)
Whited [38]	18.5 (25/135)
Eminovic [11]	42 (40/96)
Mahendran [13]	13 (21/163)
Moreno-Ramirez [20]	51 (111/219)
Knol [39]	53 (163/306)
Bowns [16]	58 (53/92)

photographs appended to a referral letter as the "teledermatology" consultation. The study by Taylor et al. also demonstrated the potential utility of teledermatology as a triage tool indicating that only 32% of the teledermatology referrals would have been scheduled for an urgent clinic consultation compared with 64% by the conventional consult process [9].

An outcome, although still intermediate, that is more closely linked to a patient's clinical course is the time to initial intervention or point of initial evaluation by a dermatologist. A randomized trial compared time to intervention between patients undergoing store-and-forward teledermatology consults and a conventional clinic-based consult process [38]. Time to intervention was defined as the time from referral to clinic visit (if a visit was required) or time from referral to the date the consult was answered (if a clinic visit was not required) in both study arms. Thus, teledermatology patients who required a clinic visit were not considered to have reached a point of intervention until presentation to the dermatology clinic. Patients undergoing store-and-forward teledermatology consultations reached a point of intervention significantly sooner than did patients undergoing the conventional referral process – median of 41 vs 127 days, respectively.

Another study found that store-and-forward consults were answered on average in 2.17 days which compared to an average 90-day wait for a clinic-based appointment in the university setting and an average 17.18-day wait in the local community [40].

Two studies assessed the time required by dermatologists to review a teledermatology consult. A study by van den Akker et al. found that it took dermatologists a median of 10 min to review a store-and-forward tele-dermatology consult [41]. A study by Whited et al. found that dermatologists required an average of 7.2 min to review a store-and-forward teledermato-logy consult compared to 24.4 min for clinic-based visits [42].

Real-time interactive

Only one study made an assessment of clinical improvement among patients undergoing real-time interactive teledermatology consultations [43]. The outcomes of patients who underwent two teledermatology consults were retrospectively reviewed. Of 127 subjects reviewed, 74 (58.3%) were rated as showing "clinical improvement," 21 (16.5%) were rated as showing "no clinical improvement," 9 (7.1%) were rated "not compliant," and 23 (18.1%) were rated "not applicable." Not applicable implied the patient had a chronic condition that would not be expected to change. The study did not include a control group of patients undergoing conventional clinic-based consults.

Real-time interactive teledermatology has been more successful in avoiding dermatology clinic visits. Reports in the literature range from 44.4% to 82% of clinic visits averted.

Five studies that have evaluated the proportion of real-time interactive teledermatology consults that avoided a clinic-based visit to a dermatologist appear in Table 4-10.

Three studies have compared the time required to perform real-time interactive consultations vs clinic-based care from both the patients' and dermatologists' perspectives. The patient perspective included travel considerations and waiting times. In a study by Loane et al. [48] total consult

Table 4-10: Dermatology clinic visits avoided with real-time interactive teledermatology

Reference	Dermatology clinic visits avoided (%)
Loane [36]	55 (53/96)
Loane [44]	44.4 (56/126)
Wootton [45]	54 (55/102)
Lamminen [46]	72 (18/25)
Granlund [47]	82 (18/22)

time from the patients' perspective was 59.3 min for real-time consults and 84.4 min for clinic-based care. Dermatologists spent 22 min performing teledermatology consults compared to 16.8 min for conventional care. A study by Oakley [49] found that patients spent 51 min for real-time consults compared to 259 min for usual care. Dermatologists spent an equal amount of time, 23 min, with both consult modalities. A final study by Loane et al. [50] found that patients required 52.6 min for real-time consults and 259 min for conventional care. Dermatologists spent 20 and 21.6 min for real-time consults and conventional care, respectively. Thus, little to no time savings are realized with real-time consults from the dermatologists' perspective.

Summary of clinical outcomes research

Clinical outcomes are one of the least researched areas of teledermatology. To date, only one study has been published that assessed a definitive clinical outcome using a randomized clinical trial design that indicated comparable clinical outcomes. Assessments of intermediate outcomes when using store-and-forward teledermatology have shown that approximately one in four teledermatology consults do not require a clinic-based visit, in settings where clinic-based care was normally available. A greater proportion of real-time interactive consultations avoid the need for a clinic-based evaluation (approximately 50%); however, time requirements to perform these consultations are similar to the time required to perform clinic-based evaluations.

Economic analyses

Interpretation of economic analyses depend on two main factors. The first is the type of economic analysis undertaken (for example, that is cost-effectiveness analysis, cost-benefit analysis). The second is the economic perspective taken by the analysis. In general, the societal economic perspective is considered the most relevant since it is an attempt to account for all the costs and outcomes encountered with an intervention. However, payers of healthcare services, such as government agencies and managed care organizations, are often interested in their own perspective. Expenditures that their organizations incur may be of greater interest to them than those costs that accrue, for example, by patients or employers for loss of work, productivity, or travel. Thus, assessment of perspectives other than a societal perspective are also important.

Store and forward

Very little information is available regarding the economic impact of store-and-forward teledermatology. A study by Whited et al. found that, from the

Table 4-11: Economic analyses of real-time interactive consult modalities

Reference	Analysis	Consult cost by modality		Perspective	Setting
		Real Time	Conventional care		
Wootton [45]	Cost-benefit	£132.10 (per patient)	£48.73 (per patient)	Societal	Community care
Loane [44]	Cost-benefit	£146.48 (per patient)	£47.3 (per patient)	Societal	Urban community care
	Cost-benefit	£180.22 (per patient)	£48.77 (per patient)	Societal	Rural community care
Lamminen [46]	Cost	18,627 FM (total cost)	18,034 FM (total cost)	Societal	Community care
Bergmo [51]	Cost-minimization	NKr 470,780 (total cost)	NKr 635,075 (total cost)	Healthcare sector	Community care
Loane [50]	Cost-minimization	NZ $279.23 (per patient)	NZ $283.70 (per patient)	Societal	Rural community care
Chan [52]	Cost	HK $57.7	HK $322.8	Healthcare sector	Institutionalized patients
Persaud [53]	Cost-minimization	Can $619.02–4,163.09 (per patient)	NA[a]	Societal	Community care

Note: [a] Average costs for conventional care not reported. Total costs for real-time consults (that included psychiatry consults) ranged from Can $1,736 to $28,084 and for conventional care ranged from Can $325 to $1,133.

Department of Veterans Affairs' economic perspective, store-and-forward teledermatology was the more costly alternative, costing an average of $36.40 per teledermatology patient compared to $21.40 for patients undergoing conventional consults [42]. However, when the societal economic perspective was taken, store-and-forward teledermatology did become a cost-saving strategy. Despite its greater costs, store-and-forward teledermatology was a very cost-effective strategy for the Department of Veterans Affairs, incurring an additional $0.17 per patient per day of time to intervention saved. A study by Zelickson et al. suggested that store-and-forward teledermatology would be a cost-saving strategy when used in a nursing home facility, although a formal cost-effectiveness analysis was not performed [5].

Real-time interactive

Much more research has been performed on the economic impact of real-time interactive teledermatology. Several well-designed studies have assessed the economic impact of real-time interactive teledermatology consult systems and are summarized in Table 4-11. Results have run the gamut from real-time technology being the more costly alternative to cost neutrality to cost savings. All existing studies have focused on the cost side of the ratio, with no studies performing cost-effectiveness analyses.

An additional study that used economic modeling by Lamminen et al. found that real-time interactive teledermatology could be cost saving, but was volume dependent [54]. That is, consult volume could be used to predict the economic outcome. Existing studies serve to illustrate the point that various factors, such as the economic perspective or setting and other patient-related factors, often influence the economic outcome.

Summary

The economic impact of store-and-forward teledermatology is inconclusive with only one existing study that performed a cost-effectiveness analysis. This study showed that store-and-forward teledermatology was the more costly alternative from the economic perspective of the healthcare agency. However, it was a cost-effective intervention in terms of improving access to care as measured by time to intervention. This gain in effectiveness would not be realized in settings that had ready access to dermatologic care. Much more research has been performed on real-time interactive technology with mixed results. Typically, real-time interactive technology is more costly than conventional care, with several well-designed studies supporting this conclusion. However, in some settings it incurs equivalent costs or even results in cost savings. The economic perspective and setting, as might be expected, often influence the economic conclusions drawn.

Satisfaction assessments

Reliable and validated instruments to assess satisfaction among participants of teledermatology consults do not exist. The existing research primarily consists of proprietary scales that are largely anecdotal but do display some face validity. There are three main users of teledermatology consult systems – patients, referring clinicians, and consulting dermatologists. Studies have addressed the satisfaction with teledermatology of all three user groups.

Store and forward

PATIENT SATISFACTION

The major findings and themes that arise from the literature on patient satisfaction with store-and-forward technology appear in Table 4-12. In the study by Williams et al. patients were ambivalent about whether they were more comfortable using teledermatology vs a clinic visit – 40% were more comfortable with clinic visits, 42% were more comfortable with teledermatology, and 18% were neutral [55]. Likewise, in a study by Collins et al. 38% of patients preferred in-person evaluations, 32% preferred teledermatology, and 30% were unsure [56]. An additional study found that 41.5% of subjects would rather have a teledermatology consultation, 22% were neutral, and 36.5% preferred an in-person visit [57].

Referring clinician satisfaction

The major findings and themes that arise from the literature on referring clinician satisfaction with store-and-forward technology appear in Table 4-13. In a study by Collins et al. referring clinicians did not have favorable opinions of teledermatology [61]. Of note, the referring clinicians in this study were required to obtain the images, enter the referring the clinical data, and transmit the consult.

Consultant satisfaction

Few studies have made assessments of dermatologist consultants' satisfaction. Those that have appear in Table 4-14. Consultant dermatologists were less confident in their diagnoses when using teledermatology.

Real-time interactive

PATIENT SATISFACTION

The major findings from the literature on patient satisfaction with real-time interactive technology appear in Table 4-15. As with store-and-forward consults, patients expressed no strong preference for usual care vs teledermatology [23, 28, 62].

Table 4-12: Major findings from store-and-forward patient satisfaction assessments

Reference	Positive features and comments	Negative features and comments	Overall satisfaction
Weinstock [58]	75% of respondents would recommend teledermatology	Long waiting times before learning of consult results	42%
Pak [59]	39% believed teledermatology saved time	Lack of follow-up after the consult	64%
Kvedar [60]	Satisfied that concerns were addressed	NA	4.56 on a 5-point scale
van den Akker [41]	Comfortable with using digital images	Concerned about incomplete information being transmitted via teledermatology	7.4 on a 10-point scale
Williams [55]	86% were satisfied with the convenience of teledermatology	30% expressed discomfort with not speaking to a dermatologist	93%
Collins [56]	85% would be happy to use teledermatology again and 78% were satisfied with the general practitioner providing the results/treatment of the consult	40% felt something was missing by not seeing a dermatologist in person	76%
Whited [57]	84% had confidence that the dermatologist could help them by looking at images	20% rated the time required to be informed of the consult outcome as fair or poor	82%
Bowns [16]	76% would rather be managed by teledermatology than to have to wait several weeks for a clinic appointment	40% felt something important was missing if they did not see an in-person dermatologist	81%

Table 4-13: Major findings from store-and-forward referring clinician satisfaction assessments

Reference	Positive features and comments	Negative features and comments	Overall satisfaction (%)
Weinstock [58]	74% would recommend teledermatology	Consult process took too long and the backlog was too great	63
Pak [59]	Believed they received an educational benefit	NA	NA
Kvedar [60]	Would like to continue using teledermatology and found it convenient	Time requirements to generate the teledermatology consult	NA
van den Akker [41]	Believed they received an educational benefit	NA	NA
Collins [61]	Improved access to experts	Time consuming referral process, increased workload, 23% would consider using teledermatology in the future	21
Whited [57]	84% preferred teledermatology to the conventional consult process	NA	92
Bowns [16]	60% expressed aspects of teledermatology they liked	Time consuming process, increased workload, complex teledermatology system	21

Table 4-14: Major findings from store-and-forward consultant satisfaction assessments

Reference	Positive features and comments	Negative features and comments	Overall satisfaction (%)
Pak [59]	70% believed that the consult was of sufficient quality to make a diagnosis	Clinic visits would have made them more confident of the diagnosis	NA
van den Akker [41]	Image quality was good	NA	NA
Whited [57]	100% stated that triage was easier	75% were less confident in their diagnoses and management plans	75
Bowns [16]	Teledermatology system was easy to use	Lack of patient contact, less confident in diagnoses	NA

Referring clinician satisfaction

Referring clinician satisfaction assessments when using real-time inter-active technology appear in Table 4-16. A positive educational benefit was mentioned in both surveys.

Consultant satisfaction

Satisfaction among dermatologist consultants using real-time interactive technology appear in Table 4-17. As was seen with store-and-forward techniques, dermatologists expressed greater confidence with in-person examinations.

Summary

Although patient and clinician satisfaction data are anecdotal, some recurring themes emerged from the literature. Overall, patients are satisfied with receiving dermatologic care with either consult modality. Long waits for follow-up, or even lack of follow-up, have been the biggest problems identified with store-and-forward consults. Patients have expressed ambivalence about a preference for teledermatology vs usual care, suggesting that

Table 4-15: Major findings from real-time interactive patient satisfaction assessments

Reference	Positive features and comments	Negative features and comments	Overall satisfaction (%)
Reid [63]	Teledermatology is of value to patients and the community	NA	NA
Nordal [28]	Overall, reported that features of teledermatology were as good or better than clinic-based care	14% report lack of hands-on examination a disadvantage	NA
Loane [62]	66% reported that teledermatology was as good as clinic-based care	13% expressed discomfort because of the camera	NA
Gilmour [23]	59% believed teledermatology was just as good as clinic-based care	18% expressed discomfort with the camera	NA
Hicks [64]	Only 3% rated teledermatology as "not as good" as a clinic visit	NA	88

Table 4-16: Major findings from real-time interactive referring clinician satisfaction assessments

Reference	Positive features and comments	Negative features and comments	Overall satisfaction
Jones [65]	Positive educational benefit	Consults were time consuming	NA
Gilmour [23]	Positive educational benefit	Some problems with sound and visual quality reported	NA

Table 4-17: Major findings from real-time interactive consultant satisfaction assessments

Reference	Positive features and comments	Negative features and comments	Overall satisfaction
Lowitt [24]	98% believed good rapport with patients was achieved	Expressed greater confidence in clinic-based diagnoses	NA
Nordal [28]	80% believed the teledermatology examination was as thorough as clinic-based care	Expressed better contact with patient with in-person examinations	NA

they perceive either option to be an acceptable means of obtaining dermatologic care. For referring clinicians, the educational benefit they perceive as a result of the consult process is the most commonly mentioned positive feature. Time constraints involved with consult generation with both modalities is frequently mentioned as a negative aspect. Fewer studies have made assessments of the dermatologist consultants' perceptions. Overall, dermatologists have been satisfied with the consult process, but report greater confidence when making diagnoses through clinic-based visits.

Directions for future research

While teledermatology is one of the best-studied disciplines in telemedicine, there are several issues that need to be explored or further defined. Existing research that examines diagnostic reliability is fairly comprehensive. The greatest need for future research in this area is for additional studies that simultaneously examine the level of diagnostic agreement found among different clinic-based examiners so that this "baseline" level of agreement can be compared to that found between teledermatologists and clinic-based examiners and between different teledermatologists. Reproducing or refuting the results of the two existing studies that made this assessment among different clinic-based examiners is an area of need [8, 22].

Future studies that more completely describe management recommendation reliability would add to the current body of evidence that has focused on biopsy recommendations. However, because of the aforementioned limitations of management reliability research, correlating reliability data with processes of care, clinical outcomes, and economic outcomes would be most useful additions to the current body of research. Agreement on management recommendations has some usefulness, but should be considered an intermediate outcome. Different management strategies may reflect more on the preferences of particular clinicians and have little, if any, impact on clinical outcomes.

Because of the lack of a gold standard test that can be universally applied across the scope of dermatologic disease, assessments of diagnostic accuracy can be problematic, thus, highlighting the importance of reliability evaluations. Nonetheless, assessments of diagnostic accuracy when using real-time interactive technology are absent from the literature and additional accuracy studies when using store-and-forward technology would be useful to determine whether the existing data is reproducible. Studies that assess the ability of examiners to dichotomize lesions into benign vs malignant skin conditions, for which histopathologic review can act as a gold standard, should be emphasized in future accuracy studies. Forthcoming data will be available in that regard (personal communication Erin M. Warshaw, VA Medical Center, Minneapolis, MN).

Future studies that add to the sentinel study on clinical outcomes, that assess a definitive clinical endpoint are the most vital area to target for future teledermatology research. Not only is clinical course ultimately the most relevant metric to assess, it subsumes all previous features of teledermatology. Patients may receive varying management recommendations, or for that matter varying diagnostic possibilities; however, the treatment plan may result in a similar clinical outcome regardless of which modality is being assessed. Because ambulatory presentations of skin disease rarely result in mortality or significant morbidity (e.g., hospitalizations) quality of life assessments as a clinical endpoint acquire a particular relevance. Skin disease can have profound effects on the quality of life [66–69]. It is important to determine not only whether teledermatology achieves better clinical outcomes (which may be an unreasonable expectation), but also whether teledermatology patients achieve at least equivalent clinical outcomes. If teledermatology achieves equivalent clinical outcomes, not only could patients expect comparable results from teledermatology, but other benefits may also be realized such as more efficient use of limited resources or economic advantages.

Additional studies on the economic impact of store-and-forward teledermatology are warranted. The fixed and variable costs associated with store-and-forward teledermatology are usually lower than real-time interactive technology, but whether that cost advantage translates into store-and-forward teledermatology becoming a cost-saving modality compared to conventional care is largely unknown. Future studies of the economic impact of real-time technology should focus on cost-effectiveness trials. While costs have varied in the existing studies, it is unclear whether teledermatology would be considered a cost-effective strategy. That is to say, while it may be a more costly strategy, the gains in effectiveness may be considered "worth" the additional costs.

Development of a reliable and validated instrument that can be used to assess satisfaction among both patients and clinicians is the most pressing need for future satisfaction assessments. Existing studies have identified some recurring themes and issues that would serve as very useful foundations for formal instrument development. Whether the largely anecdotal evidence that suggests overall high satisfaction among all users of teledermatology can be validated in future research remains to be seen.

A review of the teledermatology literature entitled Summary of the Status of Teledermatology Research that is updated annually can be found at www. americantelemed.org/ICOT/sigtelederm.htm. This is the web site for the Teledermatology Special Interest Group of the American Telemedicine Association.

REFERENCES

[1] Sackett DL, Haynes RB, Guyatt GH, Tugwell P. *Clinical epidemiology: A basic science for clinical medicine*, 2nd edn. Boston, MA: Little Brown, 1991.

[2] Fletcher RH, Fletcher SW, Wagner EH. *Clinical epidemiology: The essentials*, 3rd edn. Baltimore, MD: Williams & Wilkins, 1996.

[3] Whited JD, Hall RP. Diagnostic accuracy and precision in assessing dermatologic disease: Problem or promise? *Arch Dermatol* 1997;133:1409–15.

[4] Kvedar JC, Edwards RA, Menn ER, et al. The substitution of digital images for dermatologic physical examination. *Arch Dermatol* 1997;133:161–7.

[5] Zelickson BD, Homan L. Teledermatology in the nursing home. *Arch Dermatol* 1997;133:171–4.

[6] Lyon CC, Harrison PV. A portable digital imaging system in dermatology: Diagnostic and educational applications. *J Telemed Telecare* 1997;3(S1):81–3.

[7] High WA, Houston MS, Calobrisi SD, Drage LA, McEvoy MT. Assessment of the accuracy of low-cost store-and-forward teledermatology consultation. *J Am Acad Dermatol* 2000;42:776–83.

[8] Whited JD, Hall RP, Simel DL, et al. Reliability and accuracy of dermatologists' clinic-based and digital image consultations. *J Am Acad Dermatol* 1999;41: 693–702.

[9] Taylor P, Goldsmith P, Murray K, Harris D, Barkley A. Evaluating a telemedicine system to assist in the management of teledermatology referrals. *Br J Dermatol* 2001;144:328–33.

[10] Lim AC, Egerton IB, See A, Shumack SP. Accuracy and reliability of store-and-forward teledermatology: Preliminary results from the St. George Teledermatology Project. *Australas J Dermatol* 2001;42:247–51.

[11] Eminovic N, Witkamp L, Ravelli AC, et al. Potential effect of patient-assisted teledermatology on outpatient referral rates. *J Telemed Telecare* 2003;9:321–7.

[12] Du Moulin MF, Bullens-Goessens YI, Henquet CJ, et al. The reliability of diagnosis using store-and-forward teledermatology. *J Telemed Telecare* 2003;9: 249–52.

[13] Mahendran R, Goodfield MJ, Sheehan-Dare RA. An evaluation of the role of a store-and-forward teledermatology system in skin cancer diagnosis and management. *Clin Exp Dermatol* 2005;30:209–14.

[14] Oakley AM, Reeves F, Bennett J, Holmes SH, Wickham H. Diagnostic value of written referral and/or images for skin lesions. *J Telemed Telecare* 2006;12: 151–8.

[15] Tucker WF, Lewis FM. Digital imaging: A diagnostic screening tool? *Int J Dermatol* 2005;44:479–81.

[16] Bowns IR, Collins K, Walters SJ, McDonagh AJG. Telemedicine in dermatology: A randomized controlled trial. *Health Technol Assess* 2006;10:1–39.

[17] Landis JR, Koch GG. The measurement of observer agreement for categorical data. *Biometrics* 1977;33:159–74.

[18] Krupinski EA, LeSueur B, Ellsworth L, et al. Diagnostic accuracy and image quality using a digital camera for teledermatology. *Telemed J* 1999;5:257–63.

[19] Baba M, Seckin D, Kapdagli S. A comparison of teledermatology using store-and-forward methodology alone, and in combination with Web camera videoconferencing. *J Telemed Telecare* 2005;11:354–60.

[20] Moreno-Ramirez D, Ferrandiz L, Bernal AP, Duran RC, Martin JJ, Camacho F. Teledermatology as a filtering system in pigmented lesion clinics. *J Telemed Telecare* 2005;11:298–303.

[21] Pak HS, Harden D, Cruess D, Welch ML, Poropatich R. Teledermatology: An intraobserver diagnostic correlation study, part 1. *Cutis* 2003;71:399–403.

[22] Lesher JL, Davis LS, Gourdin FW, English D, Thompson WO. Telemedicine evaluation of cutaneous diseases: A blinded comparative study. *J Am Acad Dermatol* 1998;38:27–31.

[23] Gilmour E, Campbell SM, Loane MA, et al. Comparison of teleconsultations and face-to-face consultations: Preliminary results of a United Kingdom multicentre teledermatology study. *Br J Dermatol* 1998;139:81–7.

[24] Lowitt MH, Kessler II, Kauffman CL, Hooper FJ, Siegel E, Burnett JW. Teledermatology and in-person examinations: A comparison of patient and physician perceptions and diagnostic agreement. *Arch Dermatol* 1998;134:471–6.

[25] Loane MA, Corbett R, Bloomer SE, et al. Diagnostic accuracy and clinical management by realtime teledermatology. Results from the Northern Ireland arms of the UK Multicentre Teledermatology Trial. *J Telemed Telecare* 1998;4:95–100.

[26] Phillips CM, Burke WA, Shechter A, Stone D, Balch D, Gustke S. Reliability of dermatology teleconsultations with the use of teleconferencing technology. *J Am Acad Dermatol* 1997;37:398–402.

[27] Phillips CM, Burke WA, Allen MH, Stone D, Wilson JL. Reliability of telemedicine in evaluating skin tumors. *Telemed J* 1998;4:5–9.

[28] Nordal EJ, Moseng D, Kvammen B, Lochen M-L. A comparative study of teleconsultations versus face-to-face consultations. *J Telemed Telecare* 2001;7: 257–65.

[29] Pak HS, Harden D, Cruess D, Welch ML, Propatich R. Teledermatology: An intraobserver diagnostic correlation study, part II. *Cutis* 2003;71:476–80.

[30] Shapiro M, James WD, Kessler R, et al. Comparison of skin biopsy triage decisions in 49 patients with pigmented lesions and skin neoplasms: store and forward teledermatology versus face-to-face dermatology. *Arch Dermatol* 2004;140:525–8.

[31] Whited JD, Mills BJ, Hall RP, Drugge RJ, Grichnik JM, Simel DL. A pilot trial of digital imaging in skin cancer. *J Telemed Telecare* 1998;4:108–12.

[32] Loane MA, Gore HE, Bloomer SE, et al. Preliminary results from the Northern Ireland arms of the UK Multicentre Teledermatology Trial: Is clinical management by real-time teledermatology possible? *J Telemed Telecare* 1998;4:3–5.

[33] Harrison PV, Kirby B, Dickinson Y, Schofield R. Teledermatology - high technology or not? *J Telemed Telecare* 1998;4(S1):31–2.

[34] Pak H, Triplett CA, Lindquist JH, Grambow SC, Whited JD. Store and forward teledermatology results in comparable clinical outcomes compared to conventional clinical clinic-based care. *J Telemed Telecare* 2007;13:26–30.

[35] Krupinski EA, Engstrom M, Barker G, Levine N, Weinstein RS. The challenges of following patients and assessing outcomes in teledermatology. *J Telemed Telecare* 2004;10:21–4.

[36] Loane MA, Bloomer SE, Corbett R, et al. A comparison of real-time and store-and-forward teledermatology: A cost-benefit study. *Br J Dermatol* 2000; 143:1241–7.

[37] White H, Gould D, Mills W, Brendish L. The Cornwall dermatology electronic referral and image-transfer project. *J Telemed Telecare* 1999;5(S1):85–86.

[38] Whited JD, Hall RP, Foy ME, et al. Teledermatology's impact on time to intervention among referrals to a dermatology consult service. *Telemed JE Health* 2002;8:313–21.

[39] Knol A, van den Akker TW, Damstra RJ, de Haan J. Teledermatology reduces the number of patient referrals to a dermatologist. *J Telemed Telecare* 2006;12:75–8.

[40] Krupinski E, Barker G, Rodriguez G, et al. Telemedicine versus in-person dermatology referrals: An analysis of case complexity. *Telemed J E Health* 2002;8:143–7.

[41] van den Akker TW, Reker CH, Knol A, Post J, Wilbrink J, van der Veen JP. Teledermatology as a tool for communication between general practitioners and dermatologists. *J Telemed Telecare* 2001;7:193–8.

[42] Whited JD, Datta S, Hall RP, et al. An economic analysis of a store and forward teledermatology consult system. *Telemed J E Health* 2003;4:351–60.

[43] Marcin JP, Nesbitt TS, Cole SL, et al. Changes in diagnosis, treatment, and clinical improvement among patients receiving telemedicine consultations. *Telemed J E Health* 2005;11:36–43.

[44] Loane MA, Bloomer SE, Corbett R, et al. A randomized controlled trial assessing the health economics of realtime teledermatology compared with conventional care: An urban versus rural perspective. *J Telemed Telecare* 2001;7:108–18.

[45] Wootton R, Bloomer SE, Corbett R, et al. Multicentre randomized control trial comparing real time teledermatology with conventional outpatient dermatological care: A societal cost-benefit analysis. *BMJ* 2000;320:1252–6.

[46] Lamminen H, Tuomi M-L, Lamminen J, Uusitalo H. A feasibility study of realtime teledermatology in Finland. *J Telemed Telecare* 2000;6:102–7.

[47] Granlund H, Thoden C-J, Carlson C, Harno K. Realtime teleconsultations versus face-to-face consultations in dermatology: Immediate and six-month outcome. *J Telemed Telecare* 2003;9:204–9.

[48] Loane MA, Bloomer SE, Corbett R, et al. Patient cost-benefit analysis of teledermatology measured in a randomized control trial. *J Telemed Telecare* 1999;5(S1):1–3.

[49] Oakley AM, Kerr P, Duffill M, et al. Patient cost-benefits of realtime teledermatology - a comparison of data from Northern Ireland and New Zealand. *J Telemed Telecare* 2000;6:97–101.

[50] Loane MA, Oakley A, Rademaker M, et al. A cost-minimization analysis of the societal costs of realtime teledermatology compared with conventional care: Results from a randomized controlled trial in New Zealand. *J Telemed Telecare* 2001;7:233–8.

[51] Bergmo TS. A cost-minimization analysis of a realtime teledermatology service in northern Norway. *J Telemed Telecare* 2000;6:273–7.

[52] Chan HHL, Woo J, Chan WM, Hjelm M. Teledermatology in Hong-Kong: A cost-effective method to provide service to the elderly patients living in institutions. *Int J Dermatol* 2000;39:774–8.

[53] Persaud DD, Jreige S, Skedgel C, Finley J, Sargeant J, Hanlon N. An incremental cost analysis of telehealth in Novia Scotia from a societal perspective. *J Telemed Telecare* 2005;11:77–84.

[54] Lamminen H, Lamminen J, Ruohonen K, Uusitalo H. A cost study of teleconsultation for primary-care ophthalmology and dermatology. *J Telemed Telecare* 2001;7:167–73.

[55] Williams TL, May CR, Esmail A, et al. Patient satisfaction with teledermatology is related to perceived quality of life. *Br J Dermatol* 2001;145:911–17.

[56] Collins K, Walters S, Bowns I. Patient satisfaction with teledermatology: Quantitative and qualitative results from a randomized controlled trial. *J Telemed Telecare* 2004;10:29–33.

[57] Whited JD, Hall RP, Foy ME, et al. Patient and clinician satisfaction with a store-and-forward teledermatology consult system. *Telemed J E Health* 2004;10:422–31.

[58] Weinstock MA, Nguyen FQ, Risica PM. Patient and provider satisfaction with teledermatology. *J Am Acad Dermatol* 2002;47:68–72.

[59] Pak HS, Welch M, Poropatich R. Web-based teledermatology consult system: Preliminary results from the first 100 cases. *Stud Health Technol Inform* 1999;64:179–84.

[60] Kvedar JC, Menn ER, Baradagunta S, Smulders-Meyer O, Gonzalez E. Teledermatology in a capitated delivery system using distributed information architecture: Design and development. *Telemed J* 1999;5:357–66.

[61] Collins K, Bowns I, Walters S. General practitioners' perceptions of asynchronous telemedicine in a randomized controlled trial of teledermatology. *J Telemed Telecare* 2004;10:94–8.

[62] Loane MA, Bloomer SE, Corbett R, et al. Patient satisfaction with realtime teledermatology in Northern Ireland. *J Telemed Telecare* 1998;4:36–40.

[63] Reid DS, Weaver LE, Sargeant JM, et al. Telemedicine in Nova Scotia: A report of a pilot study. *Telemed J* 1998;4:249–58.

[64] Hicks LL, Boles KE, Hudson S, et al. Patient satisfaction with teledermatology services. *J Telemed Telecare* 2003;9:42–5.

[65] Jones DH, Crichton C, Macdonald A, et al. Teledermatology in the Highlands of Scotland. *J Telemed Telecare* 1996;2(S1):7–9.

[66] Finlay AY, Kahn GK, Luscombe DK, Salek MS. Validation of the Sickness Impact Profile and Psoriasis Disability Index in psoriasis. *Br J Dermatol* 1990;123:751–6.

[67] Lundberg L, Johannesson M, Silverdahl M, Hermansson C, Lindberg M. Quality of life, health-state utilities and willingness to pay in patients with psoriasis and atopic eczema. *Br J Dermatol* 1999;140:1067–75.

[68] Mallon E, Newton JN, Klassen A, Stewart-Brown SL, Ryan TJ, Finlay AY. The quality of life in acne: A comparison with general medical conditions using generic questionnaires. *Br J Dermatol* 1999;140:672–6.

[69] Kent G, Al'Abadie M. Psychologic effects of vitiligo: A critical incident analysis. *J Am Acad Dermatol* 1996;35:895–8.

5 Policies, barriers, and other issues

Joseph C. Kvedar, Karen Rheuban, and Karen E. Edison

Introduction

A steady progression toward telemedicine-enabled care has been evident for several years. Telemedicine activities within the Department of Veterans Affairs, the U.S. Military, the Indian Health Service and public and private payers and providers are all progressing independently at various speeds and in various forms.

Given clinician shortages, an aging population, a national consciousness on healthcare affordability and quality, the ubiquity of high quality and affordable telecommunication infrastructure, we are at the beginning of an inflection point of increased activity and progress in the march toward telemedicine. This is evident in a variety of ways; here are three examples:

1. At a symposium on the accelerating use of communication technologies convened at the Conference Center at Harvard Medical in 2005, James Mongan, MD, president of Partners HealthCare System, remarked, "it is inconceivable to imagine the future of healthcare without a heavy reliance on telemedicine-related products and services." More importantly, Dr Mongan identified telemedicine activities as among the institutional priorities of Partners HealthCare, the healthcare system formed by Brigham and Women's Hospital and Massachusetts General Hospital, both leading Harvard Medical School teaching hospitals.
2. In May 2006, the Health and Human Services Department's Office for the Advancement of Telehealth (OAT) issued a request for grant applications for the formation of four regional telehealth resource centers and one national telehealth resource center. This grant program is designed for mature, successful telehealth programs to assist start-up and nascent programs in their development and to provide a resource to existing programs in the implementation of more effective and sustainable telehealth services. The purpose of the regional centers is to assist healthcare organizations, healthcare networks, and healthcare providers in the implementation of cost-effective telehealth programs to serve rural and medically underserved areas and populations.

The national telehealth resource center will focus on legal and regulatory telehealth issues. Awards were granted in September 2006.

3. In June 2006, 22 world-class technology companies, consumer electronics companies and healthcare systems came together to launch Continua Health Alliance, a not-for-profit alliance of technology, medical device, and healthcare industry leaders dedicated to making personal telehealth a reality by bringing together standards and diverse technology for the consumer market. Within the first 3 months of its launch, the Continua Health Alliance corporate membership has grown more than 50%.

These three examples, all independent of one another and among many that could have been cited, evidence the coalescence of a movement in healthcare. It is inconceivable to imagine our healthcare system without integrated telemedicine-related services. For researchers, legal scholars, and policy makers, there is much to be sorted out as innovation and novel disruptive technologies and processes promise to help reengineer the care delivery process and open up new avenues of medical communication, connectedness, and interaction, all in the name of quality, efficiency, convenience, and value. This is an exciting and interesting time in medicine as a plethora of legal and regulatory issues relating to the intersection of medicine and technology come to the fore – for dermatology and for other clinical specialties – and are discussed, debated, and decided. In this chapter, we look at these issues.

Terminology and vocabulary

As a starting point, it would be reasonable to ask, What is teledermatology? Is it a product? Is it a service? Is it a real-time activity? Is it nonreal time? Is it physician-to-patient? Is it physician-to-physician? Is an intermediary involved? Does it occur in the provider setting? Does it occur outside of the provider setting? Despite the fact that these questions cover a wide range of possibilities, the answer to all of them is "yes, teledermatology is all of those things and occurs in all of those ways."

Certainly, the term "teledermatology" is subsumed in the broader term "telemedicine," which the American Telemedicine Association (ATA) defines as "the use of medical information exchanged from one site to another via electronic communications to improve patients' health status." The ATA describes videoconferencing and the transmission of still images as telemedicine modalities. Other definitions of telemedicine exist. A universal, or even domestic, consensus on the definitive meaning of the term is lacking. The ATA definition, however, is descriptive, comprehensive, and, given the broad national representation of its membership, is probably closest to a de facto national definition.

Telemedicine and teledermatology are nascent fields. To date, there has not been a need to refine the definitions to greater specificity. As the fields develop, for reasons of reimbursement, risk management, licensure, privacy, and the like, there will be a need to clarify the various types of telemedicine and teledermatology activities occurring. Surely,

1. various federal and state government grant, contract, reimbursement, and regulatory activities;
2. the ATA through its mission of advocacy and education;
3. Continua Health Alliance through its commitment to making personal telehealth a reality;
4. payer and provider organizations responding to the changing marketplace and demands of patients; and
5. the activities and interests of other stakeholders in this field

will inevitably spur national dialogue and foster collaborations that will bring about the vocabulary and terminology clarity necessary to help organize these fields further and propel them forward.

Market size

On its web site (www.americantelemed.org), the ATA reports "[a] Medicare program supporting videoconference-based patient services in non-metropolitan areas is rapidly growing but will reimburse less than $1 million this year."

Although there are no published statistics on the size of the teledermatology market, it can be taken as a given that in these early days of teledermatology the market is small. The ability to capture hard data on where teledermatology is occurring is handicapped by the present reimbursement coding structure – on its web site, the ATA reports that "in the reimbursement fee structure, there is usually no distinction made between services provided on site and those provided through telemedicine and often no separate coding required for billing of remote services." Because of the lack of coding and tracking of teledermatology activity, we have attempted to obtain utilization information by proxy. The OAT 2004–5 Grantee Directory states that OAT supports 34 teledermatology programs occurring in 25 different states. This would represent the minimum number of active teledermatology programs occurring as presumably other non-OAT funded programs exist and are not captured in the OAT Grantee Directory. (For more information on teledermatology utilization, see Chapter 3.)

An enduring attribute of teledermatology, and for that matter of all telemedicine activities, is that they have always been about creating access and connectedness. Those active in the teledermatology (and telemedicine) field have long recognized in public forums the importance of the time-honored and traditional face-to-face clinical encounter in which the physician physically examines the patient and discusses the ailment, the diagnosis, and the treatment recommendations personally. As the field matures, patients, providers, and policy leaders will refine the teledermatology process.

As this occurs, the importance of the physician-patient relationship, which is so very private, personal, and time and tradition honored, should remain unaffected and even strengthened through telemedicine connectedness.

Given the need to provide dermatological care for the broad spectrum of dermatological conditions that can affect 300 million Americans, introducing teledermatology solutions to build clinical capacity and efficiency and to enable, for example, adjunctive remote follow-up care when clinically appropriate, are all areas ripe for research and policy development. Questions of whether these research activities should be publicly or privately funded, whether they should be centrally coordinated and how teledermatology priority areas are determined are additional policy questions that will be sorted out gradually as the market matures and the various factors that bring about change – reimbursement, technology innovation, and the like – come into alignment. Organizations such as the American Academy of Dermatology and the ATA are good resources for ongoing policy considerations on these matters.

Reimbursement

Perhaps the single largest barrier to widespread adoption of telemedicine and teledermatology is the lack of a consistent broad-scale payment model that is sufficient to enable clinicians to build a sustainable telepractice.

Currently, teledermatology reimbursement arrangements vary widely depending upon the payer, provider, geography, and teledermatology business relationship and process involved. There are many areas where dermatologists are not offering teledermatology services at all. It is fair to say that the average consumer of healthcare services is largely unaware of possible telemedicine and teledermatology alternatives, if any, available to him or her. In instances where teledermatology is practiced, the teledermatologist seeks reimbursement from a governmental payer, a private payer, or the patient. A nontraditional reimbursement model may include situations where the hospital facility in which the patient is located acts as payer and reimburses the teledermatologist who then bills a government payer, a private payer, or the patient, as applicable. In still other situations, a membership fee reimbursement model is in place.

Private payer reimbursement

In 2002, the ATA and AMD Telemedicine conducted a private payer survey, which can be viewed at www.amdtelemedicine.com/private_payer/index. cfm. In summary, it found that over 100 private payers currently reimburse for telemedicine services. Since the survey was intended to be a sampling only and not an exhaustive compilation of telemedicine-related reimbursement policies of every private payer in the nation, the survey sponsors concluded that over 100 private payers identified were only a partial listing of private payers reimbursing for telemedicine services.

Federal and state government reimbursement efforts

Medicare reimburses for live-interactive patient services, including teledermatology, in nonmetropolitan areas at the same rates at which it reimburses for traditional face-to-face dermatology visits. Additionally by government mandate, store-and-forward telemedicine encounters (including teledermatology encounters) that are part of telemedicine demonstration projects in Alaska and Hawaii are reimbursed, also at the same rates at which Medicare reimburses for traditional face-to-face visits. In metropolitan areas, Medicare does not reimburse for any telemedicine or teledermatology services, regardless of whether such services are live-interactive or store-and-forward in nature.

On its web site (www.cms.gov), the Centers for Medicare and Medicaid Services (CMS) states that CMS has not formally defined telemedicine for the Medicaid program and Medicaid law does not recognize telemedicine as a distinct service. Nevertheless, Medicaid reimbursement for services furnished through telemedicine applications is available, at a state's option, as a cost-effective alternative to the more traditional ways of providing medical care (e.g., face-to-face consultations or examinations). The CMS web site reports that at least 18 states are allowing reimbursement for services provided via telemedicine for reasons that include improved access to specialists for rural communities and reduced transportation costs.

In their private payer survey results, the ATA and AMD Telemedicine reported that as of 2002, Louisiana, California, Oklahoma, Texas, and Kentucky had all passed legislation mandating private payer reimbursement for telemedicine services. They provided summaries of sample telemedicine reimbursement language as follows:

California: The act prohibits health insurers from requiring face-to-face contact between a healthcare provider and patient for services appropriately provided through telemedicine, subject to the terms of the contract.

Kentucky: Prohibits Medicaid and private insurers from excluding services from coverage solely because the service was provided through telehealth.

Oklahoma: Provides that healthcare plans cannot deny coverage for healthcare services provided through audio, video, or data communications. This would allow, for example, compensation for patient consultations, diagnoses, and the transfer of medical data through telecommunications technology. The measure excludes telephone and facsimile communications from the term telemedicine.

Texas: Prohibits certain health benefit plans from excluding a medical service solely because the service is provided through telemedicine. Telemedicine services may be subject to deductible, copayment, or coinsurance requirements not to exceed requirement for the same face-to-face services.

Modifications in this area of the law continue to occur. For example, effective May 1, 2006, the Indiana Medicaid began reimbursing providers for offering telemedicine services.

Reimbursement policy considerations

It is clear from the summary above that the reimbursement landscape for teledermatology is a patchwork of (a) nonexistent coverage and payment, (b) geographically limited governmental coverage and payment, (c) modality limited governmental coverage and payment, and (d) a variety of coverage and payment commutations and permutations among private payers. In the name of patient care quality, efficiency, convenience, and value, there is a compelling need to bring order to this mélange.

A February 2001 evidence report prepared for the Agency for Health-care Research and Quality (AHRQ) by the Oregon Evidence-Based Practice Center under contract No. 290-97-0018 stated that "teledermatology is the most-studied clinical specialty in store-and-forward telemedicine; its diagnostic accuracy and patient management decisions being made are comparable to those of in-person clinical encounters. It may improve access to care and have adequate patient acceptance." But, it states that more research and rigorous trials are needed [1].

A February 2006 evidence report prepared for the AHRQ by the Oregon Evidence-Based Practice Center under contract No. 290-02-0024, intended as an update to the 2001 evidence report, reaches largely the same conclusion and states "it appears that the expense and time commitment of teledermatology systems have not yet demonstrated the potential for improving access to care" and "in general, advocacy for an expanded role for teledermatology will require further studies that examine rates of missed diagnoses, incorrect treatments, and when the technology is insufficient to avoid in-person encounters." In the conclusion section of the report's discussion on efficacy, it states "the promise of telemedicine is not matched by the strength of its evidence base" and "there is mixed evidence for the efficacy of telemedicine in dermatology" [2].

Despite cautionary tones, the 2006 reports also states "the role of telemedicine most likely to demonstrate value could be as an adjunct to care that is centered around the in-person visit" and "telemedicine is widely used, with increasing numbers of health care payers reimbursing for its use."

Given the millions of dollars that OAT has invested in telehealth, including the recently established national and regional telehealth resource centers, and comparing that to the overall conclusions of the two evidence reports above, the government policy direction with respect to telemedicine and teledermatology can be analogized to "one foot on the gas pedal and one foot on the brake."

Further confounding the situation is the CMS web site statement, mentioned above, that at least 18 states reimburse for telemedicine services for reasons that include improved access to specialists and reduced transportation costs. Certainly, urban dwellers have a need for improved access to specialists and reduced transportation costs just as well as rural dwellers. Equally confounding are that the CMS Chronic Care Improvement Program and Care Management for High Cost Beneficiaries Program, announced over the last couple of years; both call for the use of information technology, including telemedicine, to aid in achieving program goals. Additionally, even the president through the formation of the Office of Health Information Technology has expressed a national will toward increased use of communication technologies in healthcare. Against the backdrop of all of this, the government has yet to provide funding to support the requisite research called for in both the evidence reports. Further, it has not provided a definitive path to reimbursement for private sources that might otherwise seek to commission such research programs. For telemedicine and teledermatology to reach its full potential there is a compelling need for the government to provide greater assistance and direction in this critical area.

With the vast amounts of remote electronic commerce that occurs daily in all sectors of the economy and with healthcare representing such a large and growing percentage of our economy, from a policy perspective, it is challenging to muster a rational defense of the federal government's geographic (metropolitan vs nonmetropolitan) and modality (live-interactive vs store-and-forward) restrictions on telemedicine and teledermatology. These artificial restrictions should be removed, thereby enabling the possibility of greater telemedicine and teledermatology commerce and potentially accelerating privately commissioned research studies addressing areas called for in the evidence reports.

There is indeed much to be sorted out in the telemedicine and teledermatology reimbursement arena and there is a need for recurring, direct and pointed dialogue, and debate among all stakeholders. The law, at both the federal and state levels, continues to evolve and it can be inferred that the evolution will occur at an increasingly rapid pace. More information on the evolving area of telemedicine and teledermatology reimbursement may be found in Chapter 7 and at the following web sites:

1. the ATA (www.atmeda.org), since 1993 the leading membership-based national resource and advocate promoting access to medical care for consumers and health professionals via telecommunications technology;
2. OAT (www.hrsa.gov/telehealth), formed in 1998 as a division of the U. S. Department of Health and Human Services Health Resource Ser-

vices Administration, whose responsibilities include administering federal telehealth grants, evaluating telehealth programs, and developing telehealth policy;

3. the Center for Telehealth and E-Health Law (CTeL) (www.ctel.org), a not-for-profit organization created in 1995 focused on overcoming legal and regulatory barriers to the utilization of telehealth and related e-health services; the National Telehealth Law Center at CTeL (www.telehealthlawcenter.org), an OAT funded national center whose purpose is to provide information about the legal and regulatory barriers to the expansion of telehealth; and

4. the Telemedicine Information Exchange (www.tie.telemed.org), a National Library of Medicine-funded web page that offers comprehensive information on telemedicine.

Telecommunications

The incorporation of telehealth technologies into integrated systems of healthcare offers tools with great potential to address the challenges of access, specialty shortages, and changing patient needs both in the rural and urban setting. The federal government has invested enormous funding in telehealth infrastructure and research, and yet, paradoxically, the sustainability of these telehealth programs is at issue because of statutory and regulatory barriers to the fullest implementation of advanced technologies applied to healthcare.

Further, with the April 27, 2004, Executive Order establishing the Office of National Health Information Technology Coordinator has come the mandate to develop a "nationwide interoperable health information infrastructure" to

a) ensure that appropriate information to guide medical decisions is available at the time and place of care;
b) improve healthcare quality, reduces medical errors, and advance the delivery of appropriate, evidence-based medical care;
c) reduce healthcare costs resulting from inefficiency, medical errors, inappropriate care, and incomplete information;
d) promote a more effective marketplace, greater competition, and increased choice through the wider availability of accurate information on healthcare costs, quality, and outcomes;
e) improve the coordination of care and information among hospitals, laboratories, physician offices, and other ambulatory care providers through an effective infrastructure for the secure and authorized exchange of healthcare information; and
f) ensure that patients' individually identifiable health information is secure and protected.

The development of such systems of care requires a fully deployed broadband infrastructure that includes both rural and urban America. The vision of Congress to speed the deployment of affordable broadband services though the act and its statutory provisions for universal service through the Rural Healthcare Support Mechanism has not yet been fully realized.

In the Telecommunications Act of 1996, Congress anticipated the continued modernization of telecommunications technologies and authorized the Federal Communications Commission (FCC) to revisit the services covered under the provisions of the Universal Service Fund. Since the passage of the Telecommunications Act, the FCC has issued several rulemakings regarding the Rural Healthcare Support Mechanism designed to expand the program. Yet, these rulemakings still fall short, in part because of restrictive statutory language.

Specific policy issues related to Universal Service Fund for Rural Healthcare Providers include

1. *Contributions to the fund*: Currently, by statute, only telecommunications providers contribute to the Universal Service fund. The base of that fund has decreased with the advent and deployment of newer communications services such as Voice Over Internet Protocol and greater utilization of what was previously defined as an information service. A newer paradigm of "communications service" would expand the pool of contributions to the fund.

2. *Eligible services*: Currently only telecommunications services are eligible for the highest level of discounts provided through the Rural Healthcare Support Mechanism. Information services are discounted on a percentage basis, which generally fall considerably short of telecommunications discounts. Changes in modern communications technologies (mobile, satellite, ISDN, DSL, T1, cable, modem, etc.) have blurred the distinction between telecommunications and information services such that the mechanism of connectivity is transparent to the end user.

3. *Eligible healthcare providers*: By statute, six categories of healthcare providers are eligible to receive discounts, and only when located in a rural area. It has been recommended that additional providers be considered eligible, such as nursing homes, skilled nursing facilities, hospice providers, dialysis facilities, emergency medical service providers, and certain school-based clinics. In addition, the definition of rural remains restrictive and with the newest FCC Report and Order may reverse the eligibility of previously eligible and worthy rural consult origination sites.

Addressing the specific challenges listed above, Congress and the FCC have a unique opportunity to more fully implement the vision of the Congress and the Presidential Executive Order of 2004 to improve access to healthcare for all Americans, and to facilitate the nationwide implementation of interoperable health information technologies to reduce medical errors, improve quality, and produce greater value for our health-care expenditures.

Licensure

One of the essential attributes of telemedicine is facilitating a clinical interaction between two geographically separated individuals. What happens when the geographic distance between the two crosses state lines?

The practice of medicine, which includes diagnosing, treating, or prescribing, is regulated at the state, not federal, level. Accordingly, each state has its own procedures for granting an individual the right to practice medicine within its borders. This restriction has often been cited as a barrier to the adoption of telemedicine. Surely, to be licensed to practice medicine in more than one state a physician would have to complete the necessary paperwork, pay the fees, and otherwise fulfill the licensure requirements of each state in which the individual seeks to become licensed. Most physicians would find this process time consuming and prohibitively expensive. Undoubtedly, only a relative few would find the process as within their economic interest.

As an exception to the practice-of-medicine laws, most state medical practice laws permit out-of-state physicians to engage in consultation with in-state physicians. It is clear, however, that whenever a physician has a direct interaction with a patient, the physician should be licensed in the state where the patient is located at the time of the interaction. State exceptions vary and should be carefully reviewed and understood prior to engaging in any activity that could potentially be determined to be practicing medicine without a license.

Many telemedicine proponents have made compelling arguments that the various state medical licensure laws have not kept up with technological advancements, that they are anticonsumer statutes designed to protect local healthcare providers, and that for our modern and mobile society to achieve full utility of telemedicine technology the ability to practice medicine across state lines is essential. Further, to stimulate discussion and generate dialogue, they have proffered a variety of possible licensure models. States, on the other hand, view their medical licensure laws as consistent with their responsibility to protect the health and welfare of their citizens against unscrupulous and incompetent practitioners. They point out that under the current process they can validate the credentials of all doctors who are licensed in their state and can hold them accountable.

Undoubtedly, the interstate licensure laws have had some impact on the slow growth and adoption of telemedicine and teledermatology. In-state telemedicine and teledermatology clinical encounters occur, but these are nowhere near the point of a clinical culture shift and a change in the practice of medicine. Thus, it is questionable how much the growth of these fields has been stymied as a result of interstate licensure barriers. Until the reimbursement issues mentioned above are resolved in a manner favorable to a telemedicine-enabled care process, it is unlikely that a relaxation of the current interstate licensure laws would have any meaningful effect on the growth of telemedicine. For policy-oriented individuals following this field, it would seem that this issue should be monitored but is, perhaps, a secondary priority focus area. The Federation of State Medical Boards, the ATA, OAT, CTeL, and TIE are all useful resources of information for those interested in monitoring developments in this area.

Malpractice and other liability risks

To prevail in a medical malpractice case, a plaintiff must prove that (a) a physician-to-patient relationship existed, (b) a standard of care was breached, and (c) an injury resulted.

To date, no case of telemedicine malpractice has been reported. As telemedicine interactions grow, undoubtedly this will change. Several issues will arise.

1. Was a physician-to-patient relationship established? When? Where? How?
2. Was there a breach of a standard of care? What standard? Is it higher than, equal to, or less than the standard of care due for physicians practicing traditional face-to-face medicine? In seeking a telemedicine interaction did the patient assume the risk of a lower standard of care?
3. In the case of interstate telemedicine activities, in what jurisdiction – the location of the patient or the location of the physician – can the lawsuit be filed? What law will govern and how will disputes be resolved?

In addition to licensure issues, there are breach of confidentiality, breach of contract, fraud and abuse, hardware, software, and telecommunications link failure risks, and potentially various other federal and state statutory and common law liability risks to evaluate and mitigate. Telemedicine and teledermatology interactions occur every day. Risk evaluation and mitigation occur through internal discussion, contracting party negotiations, purchase of adequate insurance coverage, disclosure and patient informed consent, the development of processes and protocols, redundant back up systems and staff training. Thus, while these are all important issues to address and at the outset can seem overwhelming and even extraordinarily complicated, they have not been an impediment to the telemedicine activities occurring throughout the country every day. Legal counsel is available to offer assistance. There are various conferences throughout the country that focus on these topics and the soon-to-be inaugurated regional and national telehealth resource centers should help to provide direction and clarity. As the field matures, various user or provider interest groups will undoubtedly develop broader policy pronouncements to help bring about greater efficiencies and uniform process standards.

Credentialing and privileging

Physicians engaged in the provision of telemedicine and teledermatology services must comply with state credentialing and privileging rules. In instances where organizations certified by the Joint Commission on Accreditation of Healthcare Organizations (JCAHO) participate in the provision of the telemedicine or teledermatology service, it will also be necessary to adhere to JCAHO standards.

State credentialing requirements are not identical throughout the United States. Thus, for each telemedicine relationship contemplated, the relevant state requirements must be reviewed.

Physicians providing clinical care to patients via a live-interactive link are subject to JCAHO credentialing and privileging at the site from which they are providing care (this is known as the "distant site"). The site where the patient is located (known as the "originating site") may use the credentialing and privileging information from the distant site if

1. the distant site is JCAHO accredited;
2. the physician has privileges at the distant site for the services provided at the originating site; and
3. the originating site has evidence of an internal review of the physician's performance of these privileges.

Physicians who render care using store-and-forward systems are considered consultants and as such are not required be credentialed at the originating site.

The credentialing process is time consuming and documentation intensive, particularly for rural and underserved organizations that seek access to and support from geographically distant clinical resources. A simple uniform standard that minimized the time-consuming and document-intensive process is needed. Indeed, JCAHO standards have been revised recently to move toward that goal. It seems likely that these standards will continue to be refined, thereby minimizing the compliance effort and administrative burden while holding strong to the spirit of the standard and the requirement.

Privacy and confidentiality

State and federal laws, including the Health Insurance Portability and Accountability Act (HIPAA), were enacted to ensure confidentiality and privacy of patient information. Telemedicine encounters, just like traditional face-to-face encounters need to comply with these rules. In the context of telemedicine, there may be unique compliance issues to consider. These may include, for example,

1. an increased concern for patient privacy, especially where patient visits are occurring in real time via videoconferencing in which outsiders or

nonclinical persons might be present to facilitate the videoconferencing activities, in which the event might be recorded and stored as a matter of routine at both the originating site and the distant site, in which an outside videoconferencing organization might be facilitating the conference, through which the telecommunication connection might be over an unsecure line, and so on;

2. clarifying to whom a Notice of Privacy Practices must be given;
3. a more complicated patient consent process and authorization to use protected health information, whether the telemedicine interaction can be via videoconferencing or via store-and-forward modalities;
4. evaluating whether third parties involved in the telemedicine interaction constitute "covered entities" and as such must assume certain privacy and security obligations in order to participate in the interaction.

Conclusion

We end this chapter where we started. A steady progression toward telemedicine-enabled care has been evident for several years. We are at the beginning of an inflection point of increased activity and progress in the march toward telemedicine. For a variety of reasons, it is inconceivable to imagine our healthcare system without a heavy reliance on telemedicine-related services. For researchers, legal scholars, and policy makers, there is much to be sorted out. This, then, promises to be an exciting and interesting time as a plethora of legal and regulatory issues come to the fore and are discussed, debated, and decided. In this chapter, we looked briefly at some of those issues. As the industry develops, new issues will be raised.

REFERENCES

[1] *Telemedicine for the Medicare Population*. Summary, Evidence Report/Technology Assessment: Number 24. AHRQ Publication Number 01-E011. Rockville, MD: Agency for Healthcare Research and Quality, February 2001. http://www.ahrq.gov/clinic/epcsums/telemedsum.htm. Last accessed on August 25, 2007.
[2] Hersh WR., Hickam DH, Severance SM, Dana TL, Krages KP, Helfand M. Telemedicine for the Medicare Population: Update. Evidence Report/Technology Assessment No. 131 (Prepared by the Oregon Evidence-based Practice Center under Contract No. 290-02-0024. AHRQ Publication No. 06-E007. Rockville, MD: Agency for Healthcare Research and Quality, February 2006.

6 Business models

Hon S. Pak, Marc Goldyne, and Gail Barker

Definition

The term *business model* is relatively recent. Though it appeared for the first time in the 1950s it rose to prominence and reached the mainstream only in the 1990s. Today although the term is commonly used there is still no single dominant definition [1]. A business model is a description of how an organization functions, a general template that describes its major activities. It identifies the firm's customers and the products and services it offers. It should include a detailed plan that helps an organization assess the financial viability of the model.

Introduction

A business model also provides information about

➠ how it generates revenues and profits within a framework that brings together volume projections, associated revenue, and associated costs;
➠ the cost benefit of the model;
➠ products and services;
➠ customer markets and competition;
➠ the business process;
➠ how an organization is organized.

The process of business model design is part of business strategy, which must support the organization's mission and strategic goals.

The implementation of a company's business model into organizational structures (e.g., workflows, human resources) and systems (e.g., Information Technology architecture, production lines) is part of an organization's business operations. To this extent the creation of a business model must be consistent with the value of the organization and leadership. It must also be developed with the context of the environment (rural vs urban) and values of the customers (payers, patients, providers, employees). In simple terms, a business model describes the major stakeholders and the interrelationships.

In telemedicine, there are very few articles on business models. In fact, there is only one article on teledermatology and business models [2]. This fact may represent the immaturity of telemedicine relative to healthcare in general. However, there are some mature business models in teleradiology and emerging business models in telemental health and teledermatology. Current barriers to the development of a telemedicine business model include the state of reimbursement and licensures.

Examples of business models

1. *The Arizona Telemedicine Program (ATP)* was established in 1996 and state funding was provided to implement eight telemedicine sites. Since then the ATP has expanded to connect approximately 58 healthcare organizations representing 168 sites, using a membership-based program, formalized through legal contracts. The ATP's membership model is based on an application service provider (ASP) concept whereby organizations can share services at a lower cost [3]. The ATP acts as a virtual organization service broker and brings purchasers and providers with a common goal together. The network is open and the fee schedule is designed to be flexible enough to accommodate a variety of client needs. Any organization, non-profit or for-profit, can join. The concept is to charge a membership fee to every member based on services requested. The pricing for selected services is based on a sliding scale to ensure members only pay for those services they wish to purchase or provide. A member can contract for a turn-key operation, where the ATP provides all services, or for one or more services such as continuing education, network consultation, network connection, and training. There is also multisite discount.

The original goal of the ATP business model was to build up an equipment reserve to buffer against equipment failure, to expand the network, and to accommodate varying client needs. However, membership program income now represents approximately 30% of the ATP's total revenue.

The state of Arizona has directly benefited from the ATP membership program because telecommunications networks throughout the state have been linked. The result has been the formation of a new statewide telecommunications infrastructure. This has been accomplished at a remarkably low cost to the state because once the telecommunications infrastructure was installed, additional sites could be added by just linking a telecommunications line to the nearest connection point. The program has also provided a mechanism for various healthcare providers to either obtain or supply much-needed healthcare and education services even in remote areas of the state. Scarce clinical specialty services are now more equitably distributed to rural communities in Arizona. Equipment distributors have also been able to offer discount pricing to ATP members due to the high volume of member purchases. The membership model has worked well in Arizona, but it continues to be refined as new client demands emerge.

Their teledermatology program uses store-and-forward (S/F) technology to service this network through a subscription/membership model.
There are multiple benefits to the membership to include the specialty
network and distance learning. If a site wants to start a teledermatology
program, the program will provide training and education and connect
them to the dermatologist in their network. One of the unique characteristics of this network is that it fosters competition and encourages any
organization to join the network. The result is a more cost-effective use of
resources.

2. *University of Missouri's Telehealth Program* has been one of the leaders
in telemedicine serving rural, underserved Missourians throughout the state
since 1995. In addition to their busy teleradiology service, the Missouri
Telehealth Network provides mostly live-interactive telemedicine in 15
specialties, including teledermatology, to the rural sites. More recently they
have changed teledermatology to a hybrid technology which combines the
strengths of both S/F and live-interactive modalities. In the dermatology
clinic at the University of Missouri, teledermatology has become an integral
part of how they deliver care both in terms of workflow and business process. Several patient rooms are equipped with the necessary wall-mounted
flat LCD monitors with VTC capability. Patients seen at the referring sites
by providers are scheduled through the university dermatology clinic
scheduling office, and two half-days are set aside every week to care for
teledermatology patients from 30 rural counties. One clinic is a general
teledermatology clinic and the other a telepediatric dermatology clinic.
Reimbursement for patient visits is complete. Teledermatology care for
Medicare patients is reimbursed if the patient is in a rural county; Missouri
Medicaid pays university physicians through a pilot program with the state;
most private payers reimburse for teledermatology; the Missouri Foundation for Health provides reimbursement through a grant if the patient is
uninsured or is not eligible for other third-party reimbursement.

3. *Veterans Administration (VA) Business Model*: Given the critical short-
age of dermatologists in many, if not most, VA facilities that results in a
demand for dermatology care that often exceeds the scarce dermatology
resources, more VA's are utilizing teledermatology to improve access. The
VA is divided into many regional administrative entities called Veterans
Integrated Service Networks (VISNs). Within each VISN, the VA Medical
Centers and Hospitals often have affiliated smaller outpatient clinics called
Community Based Outpatient Clinics, many of which are in rural areas with
little if any access to specialty care. Teledermatology is used in the VA as a
means of providing dermatology care to these remote Community Based
Outpatient Clinics. Each VA region is graded based on many qualitative and
quantitative measures, which include specialty access. VA leadership holds
each VISN accountable but allows local leadership to investigate innovative
ways to improve access and quality of healthcare. Because third-party
reimbursement is a lesser issue in this setting, their main focus is to use

teledermatology as a way of improving the quality of care and access to care. Cost is not a significant driver since it is a relatively low-cost specialty with some exceptions. The VA in VISN 7 determined that earlier detection of melanoma was a significant benefit due to better access and earlier intervention by dermatologists using teledermatology. Some VA sites are using live-interactive teledermatology and some are using S/F teledermatology to improve the access to dermatologists.

In the San Francisco VA, teledermatology is used to triage and consult on new referrals and manage established patients at outpatient clinics in the local community that they would normally refer to a dermatology clinic. Most of the consults are from northern California and the Pacific Islands. This VA's business model is focused on capturing new patients for the San Francisco VA, while avoiding costly outside referrals at sites where no VA dermatologist is available. Use of teledermatology results in reduced transportation costs for patients who would otherwise need to travel to San Francisco, and encourages more efficient use of limited dermatology clinic resources. Patients are typically seen by a VA provider who then submits a consult via an electronic health record (EHR) Veterans Health Information Systems and Technology Architecture (VISTA). A nurse or a technician trained on dermatology imaging takes the appropriate images and links the images to the consult. Within minutes, the dermatologist is notified and typically answers the consult within 72 hr. The VA incorporates teledermatology into the EHR system. It is possible that as the EHR becomes more prevalent, this Health Information Technology (HIT) convergence will continue.

4. *Military at war*: At the beginning of Operation Enduring Freedom, the U.S. Army Medical Department (AMEDD) lacked a cohesive system that enabled healthcare providers to obtain expert consultation services in a deployed environment. The nature of the Professional Filler System (PROFIS) often meant providers working in a clinical setting such as emergency room physicians, oncologists, and physician assistants, who previously had easy access to colleagues in their medical treatment facility, were thrust into austere environments managing medical conditions that they may have not seen since their residency. Lacking a formal teleconsultation system, deployed providers contacted military and civilian colleagues by personal email and phones when available. Furthermore, the AMEDD had no information about the volume and types of teleconsultations, and many patients were evacuated from the theater due to lack of access to specialists.

A study of 250 evacuated from Iraq and Afghanistan primarily for a dermatologic condition over a 1-year period, from 2002 to 2003, indicated that up to 70% could have been managed by their physicians in theater if a consultative system were available. In August 2003 the Army dermatology community worked with the U.S. Army Office of the Surgeon General Office and the Army Knowledge Online (AKO) community to create a user-friendly teleconsultation system. Composed of clinicians and subject matter experts from a variety of fields, the group designed and beta tested a teleconsultation system using dermatology as the test specialty for providers in Iraq and Afghanistan. In January 2005 a formal process was introduced for the selection, fielding, and management of specialties participating in the teleconsultation program.

This teleconsultation system is based on the S/F concept using AKO as a secure email portal. Although the technology itself is not new, the "system" being described encompasses a business process, which leverages a commonly available technology in the deployed environment. The deployed provider obtains a medical history of the patient, lists the diagnosis, and attaches images. Email is routed to a group of consultants in the appropriate specialty where the on-call consultant responds with a recommendation. Teleconsultations are monitored daily and most are answered within 24 hr.

A deployed provider requesting a teleconsultation writes an email in free-text format. He or she lists as much information as necessary to obtain an expert opinion and attaches the appropriate supplements. Most emails are one or two paragraphs long. Attachments may include photographs of the patient, scanned electrocardiograms, bitmaps of x-rays, and pathology reports.

Names of the teleconsultation contact group are indicative of the specialty. Email is routed to the appropriate consultant group. Specialties may have call-team subgroups or place all of the consultants on-call at all times. The on-call consultant monitors email at work and at home. A consultant responds to the teleconsultation by pressing "Reply to All," and alerts other members of the group and the consult manager that the consultation has been answered. Other members of the group may send additional comments if warranted. The consultant may collaborate with other specialties by forwarding the teleconsultation to the distribution group. By "replying to all," consultants close the teleconsultation.

Upon receipt of the recommendation, the referring physician may either manage the patient as suggested or request additional guidance. The consult manager maintains a record of the teleconsultation making it available to the consultants if the referring physician requires assistance at a future date.

Over 90% of all consultations are answered within 6 hr from the time of receipt of the teleconsultation until a recommendation is sent. Approximately 80% of teleconsultations are answered within 3 hr of receipt. Most types of consults received to-date have included, but have not been limited to, cutaneous Leishmaniasis, ocular injuries, and burns.

More than 1,400 teleconsultations have been received from all branches of the military by over 400 healthcare providers deployed to 12 countries and U.S. Navy ships afloat in the Middle East. Over 35 evacuations were prevented for medical conditions that were managed in theater. At least eight evacuations resulted following recommendation by a consulting physician. The average cycle time is less than 7 hr from receipt of the teleconsultation until a recommendation is submitted. Consultants from all Regional Medical Commands and the majority of Army hospitals and by Air Force and Navy consultants in selected specialties participate in the program. Confirmation of many teleconsultation diagnosis have verified by in-theater pathologists and in-theater in-person specialty referrals.

Given the current asymmetric battlefield, patients minimize travel to in-theater specialists thereby avoiding serious injury from insurgent attacks. In addition, consultants assure that DoD/AMEDD protocol is promulgated and followed. The program has had very low start-up and maintenance costs. The program is scaled and can quickly adapt to fluid situations such as the deployment to Pakistan to support earthquake relief efforts or assist physicians with hurricane evacuees in Federal Emergency Management Agency (FEMA) shelters.

5. *Great Plains Army Medical Region* (GPRMC) has the most active teledermatology program in the United States. This is separate from the teleconsultation support for the soldiers deployed to the Middle East. To date, they have over 16,000 consults since its inception in 2002. There are currently over 30 sites and 500 providers all over the United States that this program supports. A Business Case Analysis showed that there were two major issues: cost of network referrals and variability in access to dermatologist (military or network) depending on the location of the military facility. The cost analysis showed that net savings from S/F teledermatology was minimal; however, the improvement in access and quality of care was significant. Therefore, a decision was made to implement this program regionwide with an initial investment by the Army medical department and sustained by the regional command that controlled the budget for the region. This program utilizes teledermatology not only as a technology but has also incorporated it in the daily workflow of healthcare delivery. It is not meant to be a replacement of the dermatologist but rather as an enabling tool to augment dermatologic care in the region. The business model includes a regular visit by a dermatologist to the referring sites in regular intervals to foster and maintain relationships and to see patients who require follow up. This focus on building relationships has allowed an evolving partnership where each is able to put a face to the technology and accelerated adoption of telemedicine.

Each referring facility has a part-time or full-time consult manager (facilitator) who manages the teledermatology consult process (imaging, history taking, and follow-up). This resource is paid for by the central program to ensure that each referring facility has access to the dermatologists virtually.

One of the most unique characteristics of this program is its incorporation of teledermatology into the residency program. Brooke Army Medical Center belongs to one of the largest dermatology residency programs in the country (21 residents). Each senior dermatology resident performs a teledermatology rotation for 1 month and sees an average of 20–30 consults each day from all over the country. The residents are given the flexibility in their schedule to complete the teleconsultations from anywhere as long as the work is done. As in a traditional residency program, each consult is supervised by the staff before the consult is sent back to the referring provider for management.

Given that the country is at war, the deployment of military physicians to include dermatologists is a reality, GPRMC has created a partnership with a university and individual dermatologists to build capacity that otherwise could not be done in a traditional sense. The shortage of dermatologists is being felt throughout the United States. This is true in both urban and nonmetropolitan areas and is exacerbated by insurance coverage limitations. GPRMC initially partnered with a few individual dermatologists to answer teledermatology consults from their home or work. The incentives were obvious since they could get reimbursed for answering consults via their computer from practically anywhere with no overhead. This partnership was expanded to the University of Miami where the staff and residents are now part of the network of dermatologists who assist in answering the consults for the GPRMC.

6. *International Model*: Partners Telemedicine Program has been using a subscription model to allow patients or organizations to pay a monthly premium to have virtual access to specialists. This offering includes the international market and is currently providing consultations to several countries as part of broader context of building partnerships with other nations. University of Nebraska has an active telemedicine program with a similar business model. The actual revenue generated from telemedicine is minimal and is considered a loss-leader. The benefits are from the relationships/partnerships that lead to patient referrals sent to UNMC for cancer treatment and other diagnostic and therapeutic reasons.

7. *Private Practice Model*: The San Francisco network that will be described is referred to as an "Open Access Model" (OAM) that allows each site in the system to communicate with any other site in the system via the Internet. Currently, the dermatologist consultants interact with 8 healthcare sites located between 100 and 250 miles from San Francisco. These are locations where medical dermatology has been designated by the State of California to be undersupplied. The referral centers consist of community health centers, regional hospitals, and private family practices. There are currently two private practice dermatologists serving as teleconsultants for the network. The basic OAM unit consists of a referral site and a consultant site each having its own uniform resource locator (URL) and utilizing digital subscriber line (DSL) connectivity for fast uploading and downloading of electronic patient files. Rather than this being "rocket science," it is essentially the description of a generic email system.

In California, the costs were compared for doing 2 years of LIV consultation to 2 years of doing S/F consultation in a private practice setting as part of a California state-sponsored telemedicine project that began in 1999 and is currently in its sixth year of operation [1]. In this urban practice, the operating costs for performing LIV consultations over a 1-year period equaled 70% of the gross reimbursement for this service. In turn, 70% of telemedicine operating costs were for use of the broadband lines; the remaining 30% went to cover the increased support for billing and scheduling personnel. The average reimbursement for a 15-min consultation was $44 (based on 94 consults), and the average overhead per consultation was $31 which led to a net reimbursement of $13. The net reimbursement rate for LIV consultations was about 25% of the average net reimbursement for an in-person office consultation and required the same amount of time; consequently, no incentive existed to incorporate LIV technology in this private practice setting in 1999.

With S/F technology, a significant portion of the overhead generated using the LIV technology was precluded. Standard Internet DSL connectivity, which is already in place for the electronic billing system, replaced the broadband ISDN lines needed for the LIV teleconsults. Also, the additional personnel costs required for traditional scheduling and billing services were no longer required because the electronic medical record software (described later) allows the provider to generate billing as part of the electronic clinical encounter. These cost savings translate into incentive for participation because the same level of reimbursement without a 70% overhead becomes acceptable. Currently, the average reimbursement rate within the network is $50 (based on 1,000 consults) and there is no significant overhead generated specifically for the S/F system because it works within the standard infrastructure of all Internet-based communication. In addition, the flexibility and convenience of the S/F system along with the ability to incorporate it into current practice ultimately led to the adoption of this teledermatology model.

A major reason for the slow adoption of S/F technology is that, until relatively recently, it has not been recognized by insurance companies as a reimbursable form of healthcare delivery. Since over 80% of current healthcare services are paid for by federal, state, or private health insurance programs, their participation is critical to the successful incorporation of S/F teledermatology as a recognized means of providing access to dermatological care.

Recently, however, as data accumulate that validate the technology, an increasing number of insurance programs have begun to provide appropriate reimbursement for S/F teledermatology. In California, Blue Cross Commercial, Blue Cross State Sponsored Programs, Health Net-Medicaid, California Public Employees' Retirement System (CALPERS) all reimburse for S/F teledermatology consults. Most recently, the California Legislature passed the Cogdill Bill (AB354) which adds S/F teledermatology and teleophthalmology to the list of consultative services that will be reimbursed by Medi-Cal (State Medicaid Program), beginning in mid-2006. This expanding participation of insurance programs creates a population of almost

5 million California citizens for whom S/F teledermatology consults will be reimbursed. In Arizona, 47 private payers as well as the state's Medicaid program have been billed and reimbursed for telemedicine services including S/F teledermatology [4].

Concepts/goals to consider when selecting a business model

The examples above are not meant to be a complete list, but rather chosen to show the various teledermatology models available and their unique characteristics. However, the successes of the programs listed above are based on some core characteristics that are common to all programs which include the following:

1. *Economically self-sustaining*: Each program above is financially self-sustaining. Although the type of reimbursements varies and may include subscription and grants, each program has figured out how to sustain its program. In reimbursement independent organizations such as DoD, VA, and self-payers such as Kaiser, a business case analysis must be done which includes both direct and indirect revenue and costs. The analysis must also include the consideration of the qualitative benefits, based on the values of the organization. An example is the military where teledermatology was started despite not being a significant cost saver, but rather due to the value placed on access and quality.

2. *Care delivery integration* (both business process and technology infrastructure): Although technology cannot be forced into a traditional workflow model, it clearly must be adapted to be minimally disruptive. The transformative power and benefit of technology are realized when technology and workflow are both customized and optimized based on the goals. University of Missouri leveraged the available technology, and selected and integrated the VTC technology into a slightly modified workflow model. This synergy was only possible due to the leadership's understanding of the impact of telemedicine and technology in healthcare arena. After years of fine tuning the adoption of teledermatology, the VTC equipment was placed in regular exam rooms and teledermatology visits were customized to resemble in-person visits in every way possible, from scheduling and billing to patient care.

3. *Improve access to or quality of care*: At the University of Miami, teledermatology is allowing them to provide access to dermatologists for the care of AIDS patients, which was not otherwise available without a long delay. The military has had tremendous success with teledermatology in using it to optimize access to the delivery of dermatologic healthcare. Through teledermatology, appropriate cases were sent to dermatology and primary care providers received valuable ongoing education and assistance in managing skin disease. This type of edu-

cation to the primary care community (who see approximately 60% of skin disease) has had a tremendous impact in healthcare in DoD. At the University of Missouri, the teledermatology program has brought access to expert dermatological care for rural and underserved patients throughout Missouri and has elevated the quality standards by providing access to a variety of dermatology subspecialists, including pediatric dermatology, to deliver this care.

Criteria to consider when selecting a business model

Selecting a business model that is right for you or your organization takes investment. It requires that you understand how you deliver care, not only in the clinical aspect but also in the business aspect. It also requires you to understand your environment and setting to include the providers and specialists in your community in addition to your patients. It should, however, start with identifying the reason you are considering utilizing or expanding a teledermatology program. The model you choose must be linked closely with the motive or the set of problems you are trying to solve.

1. *Patient demographics*: Demographics include the type of patients who would potentially be seen via teledermatology. Understanding their age, gender, and race distribution along with the type of skin conditions will help in the creation of the business model. Furthermore, the setting of patient, whether rural or urban will need to be taken into consideration for the sake of follow-up implications. Also important is the type of healthcare insurance that the patient population held by the majority of the patient population. This information will be critical in building the financial model. For example starting a S/F teledermatology program in an urban area where there is no S/F reimbursement may not be sustainable. However, in urban areas of states with Medicaid programs that reimburse for S/F teledermatology, such as Arizona, California, Minnesota, and South Dakota, this business model may make more sound financial sense.

2. *Current healthcare model*: It is critical that you understand how your organization functions. This includes the where and how patients are seen to include primary care and specialty visits. You also need to understand how the organization derives revenue and the type of expenses. A hospital that is in deficit because there is a large uninsured population may not be interested in starting a teledermatology program if they perceive that this could contribute a greater loss to their bottom line. Using a different perspective, if you can prove that teledermatology can keep patients out of the emergency room and lower costs to the organization, the interest may be significant. Thus, selling your telemedicine program could be determined by a mechanism to increase revenue (including TM as a loss leader) or as expense reduction.

3. *Technology (bandwidth)*: As mentioned above, availability of bandwidth and existing technology infrastructure will help determine the type of technology modality used in your model. In some settings where the network is available, either mode could be used. In those bandwidth limited areas, S/F may be the only option.

4. *Type of organization*: The type of organization to which you belong, whether you are a private solo dermatologist, belong to a university, or are part of a government organization, will impact your decision on the selection of a business model. The primary reason, of course, is whether you are in a closed healthcare system/self-insured where one is not reliant on third-party reimbursement (e.g., Medicaid, Medicare) or a typical Health Care Organization (HCO) where one is at least partly dependent on outside funding. Organizations such as the VA, DoD, and Kaiser Permanente are in closed systems and are more likely to start any program as long as it brings value to their patients and the organization. Other types of organizations have a more difficult time since reimbursement is variable from state to state and dependent on the patient population they are serving. Furthermore, some organizations, especially large ones, can be bureaucratic and slow to adopt changes and therefore tend not to be innovative. Smaller or medium-sized HCOs have more agility and the ability to adapt to changes in the market force. A business model, therefore, must be in alignment with the type of your organization and its values.

5. *Organization's values*: Anyone selecting a teledermatology model must understand the organization's core values and objectives. In addition, the proposed value of the teledermatology program must be consistent with the higher objectives. For example, if the hospital network is looking to expand and increase revenue, teledermatology could be presented as an opportunity to increase its outreach to more remote areas without having to hire additional dermatologists (could hire virtual dermatologists). A specific value proposition of the model must not only be consistent with the leadership's goals but must also be clearly articulated.

6. *Organizations needs/ issues (access)*: The model chosen must be consistent with the perceived needs of the organization. Regardless of how real a shortage of dermatologists is, or how long a patient has to wait to see a dermatologist, the perception of the leadership on this problem may not be consistent with your assessment of the severity. Therefore, a business model should be selected based on both real and perceived needs which have been validated by the organizational leadership. Ultimately, you will need funding and support by the leadership and selection of a business model that best fits the organization's vision and values and that solves a particular problem for the organization.

7. *Resource availability*: In the selection of the business model, one must understand the resources that are available both within the organiza-

tion and its surrounding network. This obviously includes the referring clinics or hospitals and what resources (e.g., personnel) can be utilized for teledermatology. Ideally, if there is a telemedicine facilitator at each referral center, adding a teledermatology capability would be easier. However, if there is no existing telemedicine capability, you will need to assess the adequacy of clinical staffing at the referral sites. Moreover, the model must take into consideration the capacity of the dermatologists. If your dermatologists in your network are at 100% capacity, adding the burden of teledermatology will not be well accepted. In that setting where the dermatology capacity is full, using a virtual dermatology network to the model will add significant benefit. The resource availability is not limited to personnel, since it must also include the capability of referring providers/clinics and specialists. For example, do the referring sites have the capacity to perform simple common procedures like shave and punch biopsy in addition to cryotherapy? Is there are adequate specialties, to include Moh's and dermatopathology, for the population to be served by teledermatology? Do you need to consider partnering with a local dermatologist near the referring sites to ensure that patient seen by teledermatology has adequate follow up?

Teledermatology delivery models with specific examples

Telecare

Telecare is defined as care sought by the patient and directly provided for the patient over a distance. Specifically in this delivery model, a dermatologist provides direct care to the patient by either directly interacting with a patient in real time or asynchronously (S/F). No referring provider is involved in this model.

PROS

Teledermatology provided via telecare allows patients to have direct access to a dermatologist. In states like Georgia, direct access to dermatology is mandated with the assumption (probably correct) that early intervention by dermatology will lead to faster resolution and a more accurate diagnosis. This model essentially is a goal for many in the telehealth community providing access to healthcare wherever the patient may be.

CONS

The pitfall currently with this model is that uniform standards for images acquired and cameras used are not available. Imaging protocol and training for an individual patient at home is too cumbersome. As technology improves and becomes available for the mass market, this issue will most likely disappear.

EXAMPLES

1. The best example of Telecare is live-interactive teledermatology where the patient contacts the teledermatology clinic in his or her home environment and personally initiates the visit. The initial patient care, treatment, and follow-up care are "direct" as it is in person.

2. A more indirect S/F telecare model has been shown to have promise in follow-up clinics. After a new patient has seen a dermatologist for a common skin condition such as acne or psoriasis or vitiligo, a patient takes his or her own images along with a simple questionnaire to follow up with the dermatologist online. Secure messaging systems such as Relay Health and medem are two such systems that allow this to occur, although used mostly for text information and not teleconsultation.

3. Although not currently operational, a telecare clinic could be set up in a clinic or hospice setting where a trained nurse could see patients and send the information to the dermatologist via live-interactive or S/F. The dermatologist could then contact the patient directly and manage him or her virtually.

DISCUSSION

The future of medicine is clearly going in this direction. Many want to be able to deliver care and patients want to receive this care at the patient's home or wherever the patient may be. Standards are needed, however, for an average patient to image and self-refer himself or herself for a new dermatological condition. For now, a nurse to assist in obtaining the right set of information and images or limiting it to a follow-up clinic for a specific subset of skin conditions appears to be workable.

Teletriage

Teletriage is the delivery of triage over a distance. This is being used in a very limited sense to prioritize patients and route their healthcare management depending on the triage evaluation. No diagnosis or management is performed but the evaluation is used to prioritize patient healthcare needs, determine how quickly the patient should be seen, and by whom/what clinic.

PROS

Teledermatology provided via teletriage would allow very quick and effective triage. Current methods of triage by phone or text in an EHR do not adequately provide the information necessary to perform optimal triage. Given that the access to dermatology is a significant problem in many areas of the country, teletriage would ensure that those most in need of care would receive it through a prioritized system. Enough information would be available to ensure that the right cases were being sent to the right subspecialty/procedure clinic. Some examples of this would be

⇒ Accutane Clinic
⇒ Wart Clinic
⇒ Phototherapy Clinic
⇒ Patch Clinic
⇒ Moh's/Laser/Procedure Clinic.

In certain settings the system could be used to determine whether an evacuation is needed.

CONS
The pitfall relates to the work that needs to be done at the referral sites and whether the value of the triage and optimization of resources at the central dermatology clinic justifies the cost of the workforce required at the referring clinics.

EXAMPLES
Teletriage is being done on extremely remote sites such as rigs, ships, war, airplanes, overseas, and the like.

Teletriage could be done at larger company location where a decision could be made to see if an employee needed to be seen or not.

DISCUSSION
This modality is being utilized in a very limited fashion due to the overhead cost for the referring sites. If there is already an existing infrastructure, the incremental cost may be justified. Furthermore, the burden of the quality of the information to triage but not diagnose and manage will likely be reduced. Teletriage could be used at home and as a self-referral process as long as patients are willing to pay for the convenience. As with the original model, this modality would improve access for those patients who really need care and could provide an adequate means to prioritize patients.

Telereferral

Patient is referred by a provider (physician or physician extender), but teledermatologist takes over the management limited to the skin condition.

PROS
This is most similar to the traditional referral that occurs when primary care provider is referring the patient to a specialist. The advantage of this mode is that the dermatologist is able to directly interact with the patient after the virtual evaluation for management, education, and counseling.

CONS
Most teledermatologists today prefer to provide teleconsultation rather than telereferrals. The downside of telereferral is that the referring provider

would miss the opportunity to learn from the case and manage his or her own patient.

EXAMPLES

In a site using a hybrid teledermatology system, the teledermatologist who evaluates the information and the images while the patient is present via video at the referring sites, discusses the case, educates and counsels the patient, and initiates the treatment (orders the prescription and/or tests when necessary).

In a site using S/F teledermatology, the dermatologist reviews the information and the images at a convenient time, then calls the patient at a later time to educate, discuss, counsel, and initiate treatment.

DISCUSSION

Telereferrals are being done mostly by sites using live-interactive teledermatology systems. The additional time required for the dermatologist using an S/F system to directly interact with the patient takes away some of the flexibility and the convenience for the dermatologist.

Teleconsultation

Patient is referred by a provider (physician or physician extender), and teledermatologist makes the diagnosis and recommends treatment to the referring provider. Treatment is not initiated by the teledermatologist in this model and the care of the patient is not assumed by the teledermatologist.

PROS

An analogy is the relationship between primary care and radiology. Radiologist interpret radiographs and transmit that information to primary care clinicians for their consideration and/or implementation. The radiologist does not assume the care of the patient. The advantage of this mode is that the dermatologist is able to evaluate and recommend without having to coordinate a time to talk with the patient. Most teledermatologists using S/F today prefer to do teleconsultation rather than telereferrals since the communication to the referring provider managing the patient can be done asynchronously.

CONS

The message from the dermatologist may be diluted and counseling could be suboptimal. In addition, some referring providers might not be familiar with the medications and diagnoses provided by a dermatologist. Some referring providers like the dermatologists to manage the patient instead of sending the recommendations – this may be especially true in non-incentivized settings.

EXAMPLES

Traditional teleconsultation (outpatient care – urban or rural, low volume)
Patient is seen by a provider who initiates/orders a teleconsultation. A tele-health coordinator or a nurse then obtains the information and images who submits it online. A dermatologist is notified and reviews the consult. Teleconsults could be sent from any setting as long as it was initiated by another provider.

⇒ Outpatient clinic
⇒ Inpatients at hospitals
⇒ Nursing homes.

In addition, the information is sent back as a recommendation only.

DISCUSSION

This is the most common delivery modality in sites utilizing S/F technologies. However, this does not work well in certain settings where there is only a nurse at the referral site or the referring provider does not want to manage skin diseases.

Teledermatology revenue model

There are many ways to generate revenue via teledermatology, just as in traditional dermatology. Some patients are willing to pay out of their own pockets, some have insurance, and others are grant supported. These revenue models should be evaluated and selected based on the many factors mentioned above. Below is a brief description of each type of revenue model. In most situations, you will have to select multiple revenue models.

1. *Patient self-pay/co-pay*: There is a trend toward patients' willingness to pay out of their pocket if they perceive a value for a service. For teledermatology, there has been very limited information gathering to determine if the patient is willing to pay out of pocket to be seen more quickly by telemedicine. A survey done at Partners revealed that patients were willing to pay up to $35 for improved access.
2. *Employer subsidized*: In certain locations such as a ship or a rig, some employers pay for teleconsultations, including teledermatology. In a large company with significant number of employees, some have instituted and pay for telemedicine to largely improve productivity and morale.
3. *Traditional reimbursement*: Refer to section on reimbursement.
4. *Self-insured or closed healthcare system*: In large organizations such as Kaiser Permanente, the DoD, and the VA, revenue generation is not the driving force. The issue really is one of decreasing cost via
   a) savings from referral to outside network or avoidance of contracted dermatology care

b)   savings from optimization
c)   savings from additional customers from access (market differen-
       tiator).

Many of these organizations have multiple revenue sources to include
grants, traditional third-party reimbursements, self-pay, etc. In this type of
setting, a reimbursement model is especially important to ensure that the
direct and indirect net revenue from teledermatology is positive.

1. *Indirect revenue*: In some organizations the teledermatology program
    is initiated as a loss leader since it is not costly and can facilitate the
    adoption of future advanced technology in the organization. In other
    settings, the teledermatology network is established and sustained by
    additional indirect or pull-through revenue generated from ancillary
    services and additional procedures. Examples of this include genera-
    tion of new pathology specimens, and additional referrals for more
    profitable skin surgery, cosmetics, or laser procedures. In centers such
    as University of Nebraska, which has a large cancer center, they have
    sustained and implemented a teleconsultation program with the in-
    ternational community which has led to relationships with healthcare
    organizations in various countries. Furthermore, these relationships
    have led to patient referrals for cancer and other high-cost treatments.
2. *Grants*: In most states, there are numerous grant opportunities for
    rural and urban care. Typically administered by nonprofit and gov-
    ernment organizations, these grants are available to support care for
    indigent and uninsured patients. In addition, there are many federal
    grant opportunities available such as the Office of the Advancement of
    Telehealth (OAT) which funds a variety of telemedicine programs, the
    Rural Utilities Service (RUS) which helps pay for telemedicine
    equipment, the National Library of Medicine, the Department of
    Defense, and many others.
3. *Contract reimbursement*: Dermatologists working part-time and wanting
    to supplement their income can make themselves available at a nearby
    VA, military facility, or a large primary care clinic/network. By looking
    at the ads for dermatologists, you can determine where they are having
    difficulty hiring a dermatologist. Then you can approach these organi-
    zations and ask that you do it from home. It is that simple. If you do not
    ask, you will never know. You will likely use S/F if you cannot commit to
    a regularly scheduled time, but if you can commit to some regularly
    blocked time, you could even set up a simple video teleconferencing unit
    or a webcam for a hybrid model. You could bill directly to Medicare or
    Medicaid or third party, depending on your location and patient pop-
    ulation, or you could set up a contract as did by GPRMC. If you are
    already working full time and want to supplement your income, your
    approach would be the same but limited to S/F.

What about the private practice dermatologist?

Integration of teledermatology into a contemporary medical dermatology private practice that cares for patients having multiple third-party insurance coverage plans is, at least at the present time, challenging. It is more realistic in the context of S/F technology. "Realistic" means a sustainable, low-cost program without subsidy that provides an appropriate level of reimbursement for services provided. However, as the reimbursement improves and the demand for teledermatology increases and technology continues to improve and becomes less expensive, live-interactive teledermatology could be incorporated into your practice in the future especially when combined with S/F model.

If you are semi-retiring or want to work from home or want to do only teledermatology, there are a few challenges to include generating enough volume, licensure, and malpractice insurance. Each challenge has its solution but doing teledermatology only to feed your family is a few years out. Should Medicare reimburse for S/F teledermatology, we will see a significant shift and the barriers will likely all fall with the likely formation of multiple virtual teledermatology networks.

Change in paradigm: Understanding the resource allocation and training/standards

One would look at teleradiology as a successful transition of teleradiology into our normal delivery of care. As the radiology systems became digital, the word "teleradiology" is no longer being used. It is considered "radiology." Will that happen in dermatology? Not likely given that transition of teleradiology to simply radiology represents digitalization of an interpretive specialty. Of note, the teleradiology field adopted technology standards for their specialty early on. This significantly facilitated their ability to standardize teleservices and reassure providers, patients, and regulatory agencies that care would be uniform for all patients.

In teledermatology, although the work has started in developing standards from the OAT [5], the transition is harder, especially because fundamentally, we are not an interpretive service but rather a cognitive and procedural service. Until we can automate body imaging, further develop technology standards, educate providers, patients, insurers, and regulatory agencies and it becomes affordable to automate this process, where the nurse or a telemedicine facilitator is no longer needed and EHR is able to route consultations seamlessly, the transition will likely be more gradual.

For the near future, central to the success of any telemedicine network are the personnel or "peopleware" present at the referral sites who are responsible for preparing the teledermatology visit, referral, or consultation – the so-called telemedicine site coordinators. Any group that wants to participate in the expansion of telemedicine as an effective means of healthcare delivery needs to recognize the absolute requirement of training or hiring site coordinators who are comfortable with computers and digital devices as well as having appropriate healthcare training. For dermatology, there is the additional requirement of understanding what camera and/or digital image and text data can best provide the information most germane to a teledermatologist's ability to generate an effective visit, referral, or consultation. In the Blue Cross of California Telemedicine Program, a one-page "Skin Evaluation Form" is used at the referral sites to assist the nondermatologist providers in knowing what information is needed for a dermatology S/F consult. There are other forms at the ATA web site. A standardized imaging protocol was published in the *Journal of Telemedicine and Telehealth* (JTT) last year to ensure the consistent delivery of high-quality information from the referring sites [2]. The subject of training site personnel is covered in more detail by other authors in this book. But it cannot be emphasized enough that it is the site coordinator who is the central underpinning to a successful telemedicine network because he or she insures that the camera and/or digital image and text data being provided are optimum for the teledermatologist's needs.

An evolving business model

As with any business model, it will likely evolve as reimbursement, policies, and technology change. In the last few years, a significant number of studies have been published. This includes a recently completed teledermatology outcomes study [6]. S/F teledermatology resulted in comparable clinical outcomes compared to conventional clinic-based care. We are seeing states beginning to reimburse for teledermatology. There may be a significant movement toward Medicare reimbursement and further Medicaid reimbursement in the next 1–3 years. With these reimbursement changes, the business model will evolve to focus on Medicare- and Medicaid-eligible patients for teledermatology. It is also probable that other third-party payers will be more inclined to reimburse for teledermatology services once Medicare incorporates the service into its fee schedule.

With the rise in healthcare cost there is a significant trend toward patient-centered care and patient empowerment. With this we are seeing a significant movement of energy in providing healthcare at the patient's home and on the PDA/phone. As the population ages and this aging population grows, the pressure to provide teledermatology at home will likely rise. Furthermore, as the pay-for-performance (P4P) movement matures and other performance-based incentives take hold, teledermatology and telemedicine models will also have to evolve.

Finally, technology will require us to change our models. Limitations and barriers that we cannot overcome today will no longer exist as diagnostic imaging devices (Confocal microscopy, Optical Coherence Tomography [OCT], etc.) for melanoma and other conditions become a reality and made available for providers and patients. As personal digital assistant devices/cell phones/digital cameras become more prevalent and as our population ages, healthcare and telemedicine models will have to accommodate to this reality. In the future, we will be able to perform an automated total body skin imaging and electronic and personalized health record will become common place. As these technology transformations occur, the business model for teledermatology will change, and at that point, the word teledermatology may disappear not unlike the teleradiology evolution.

Summary

In short, a business model for teledermatology is how the organization or an individual leverages teledermatology in a given setting to deliver healthcare. The context of the business model is one of sustainability, integration into the overall delivery of healthcare, and improvement of healthcare quality and access. The business models must be selected carefully and customized or adapted as illustrated for the successful programs identified in this chapter. The selection of a business model should be based on many factors but most importantly on the objectives of the individual and the organization and must be economically sustainable. Your business model will likely change and evolve with time, so selecting the perfect model the first time is not the goal.

REFERENCES

[1] Fetscherin M, Knolmayer G. Business models for content delivery: An empirical analysis of the newspaper and magazine industry. *Int J Media Manage* 2004;6(1 and 2):4–11.

[2] Pak H. Implementing a teledermatology programme. *J Telemed Telecare* 2005;11 (6):285–93.

[3] Barker GP, Krupinski EA, McNeely RA, Holcomb MJ, Lopez AM, Weinstein RS. The Arizona Telemedicine Program Business Model. *J Telemed Telecare* 2005;11 (8):397–402.

[4] Barker GP, Krupinski EA, Laursen T, Erps K, Weinstein RS. Pay per view: The Arizona Telemedicine Program's billing results. *Telemed J E Health* 2001;7(1): 287–91.

[5] Tracy J. Telemedicine technical assistance documents, a guide to getting started in telemedicine, 2004. http://telehealth.muhealth.org/geninfo/A%20Guide%20to %20Getting%20Started%20in%20Telemedicine.pdf. Retrieved October 1, 2006.

[6] Pak H, Triplett CA, Lindquist JH, Grambow SC, Whited, JD. Store and forward teledermatology results in similar clinical outcomes to conventional clinic-based care. *J Telemed Telecare* 2007;13:26–30.

7 Reimbursement models for teledermatology

Karen E. Edison and Hon S. Pak

Reimbursement for teledermatology has generally mirrored reimbursement for other forms of telemedicine. However, some states, including California, have carved out teledermatology for special reimbursement arrangements. This special treatment may be a consequence of the large body of evidence supporting the quality (e.g., interobserver diagnostic concordance) of teledermatology for the care of patients with cutaneous disease as well as the lack of access to expert dermatological care in many parts of the country (see Chapter 4). This chapter discusses the current status of reimbursement for telemedicine, including teledermatology, in the United States. Although some restrictions still apply depending on the type of payer, reimbursement for telemedicine services, including teledermatology, is increasingly common.

The early days

There was a major expansion in the use of telemedicine in the United States in the early 1990s subsidized by federal grant dollars (competitive grants and earmarks) from the U.S. Departments of Health and Human Services, Commerce, and Agriculture. The bulk of these programs were developed where a clear mission base of service and outreach exists, such as in academic health centers, or where patients are distant or otherwise expensive to transport, such as in correctional healthcare systems. Federal agencies with direct patient care responsibilities also provided substantial early investment in telemedicine. Teledermatology was a leading clinical service in the Veterans Affairs (VA) healthcare system as telemedicine was introduced to this population, and teledermatology has long been a leading clinical telemedicine service in the Department of Defense. The prominence of teledermatology in these programs was thought to stem both from the discipline's suitability (image intensive) for telemedicine and the demand for improved access to expert dermatological care.

Some states have provided start-up funds for telemedicine, usually for state university-based programs or correctional care. Private telecommunications companies have also provided seed funding across the country to telemedicine programs in hopes of demonstrating the clinical utility of their technology and communication infrastructure. While federal and state grants and private industry investments are ongoing, they are being replaced by regular sources of reimbursement for telemedicine, including teledermatology, in both the public and private sectors.

Public payers

Medicare

While Medicare has long reimbursed for interpretative services transmitted through telecommunications technologies, such as interpretation of x-rays, electrocardiograms, and electroencephalogram tapes, it has taken some time to recognize newer, nontraditional forms of telemedicine. The first sign of federal recognition of the potential of telehealth to increase access to and efficiency of healthcare was reflected in the Balanced Budget Act (BBA) of 1997. It contained legislative language that was the first step toward reimbursing telehealth services through the federal Medicare program. Beginning in January 1999, the BBA allowed physicians who examine Medicare beneficiaries to provide consultation services via telehealth and to receive payment for their services. Unfortunately, complexities in the language led to largely unworkable regulations and few claims were submitted.

In the mid- to late 1990s, the telemedicine community worked to resolve problems with the federal reimbursement rules. After much input from the telehealth community, a major expansion in Medicare reimbursement in the 106th Congress came in the form of the Medicare, Medicaid, and State Children's Health Insurance Program (SCHIP), Benefits Improvement and Protection Act of 2000 (BIPA). This legislative language led the federal agency responsible for the Medicare program (then the Health Care Financing Administration [HCFA], now the Centers for Medicare and Medicaid Services [CMS]) to issue regulations allowing for Medicare reimbursement for live-interactive telehealth if the patient is

1. located in an area designated as a rural health professional shortage area (HPSA);
2. located in a county that is not included in a Metropolitan Statistical Area (non-MSA); or
3. a patient in an ongoing federal demonstration project; and

the patient is located in

1. the office of a physician;
2. the office of a practitioner (nurse practitioner, physician assistant, clinical nurse specialist, certified registered nurse anesthetist, certified nurse midwife, clinical social worker, registered dietician, or nutrition professional);
3. a critical access hospital (CAH);

4. a rural health clinic (RHC);
5. a federally qualified health center (FQHC); or
6. a hospital.

Medicare reimbursement for the healthcare provider delivering the tele-medicine service is equivalent to reimbursement for in-person care for the same service. Eligible providers include

➠ physician
➠ nurse practitioner
➠ clinical nurse specialist
➠ clinical psychologist
➠ physician assistant
➠ clinical social worker
➠ registered dietitian or nutrition professional.

The healthcare facility where the patient is located (originating site) can bill Medicare for a telehealth facility fee. This facility fee was initially $20 and has increased by the percentage increase in the Medicare economic index (MEI) every year. Current facility fee reimbursement is $21.86 and is billed with the HCPCS code "Q3014." This may only be billed by facilities in a rural HPSA or a non-MSA county.

Medicare does not reimburse for asynchronous transmission of healthcare information followed by professional consultation, including store-and-forward teledermatology, with the exception of care delivered in Alaska or Hawaii where it is reimbursed at the same rates at which it reimburses traditional in-person visits.

CPT codes

CMS conducts an annual process designed to review proposed services for addition to or deletion from the list of services eligible for Medicare reim-bursement. Requests for adding services must be submitted by December 31 in order to be considered for the annual physician fee schedule proposed rule which is customarily published the following summer. The final phy-sician fee schedule with accepted changes is published on November 1 [1].

This annual review process has been used successfully to expand the list of services reimbursed. The list now includes

➠ professional consultations (CPT codes 99241–99255)
➠ office visits (CPT codes 99201–99215)
➠ individual psychotherapy (CPT codes 90804–90809)
➠ pharmacologic management (CPT code 90862)
➠ psychiatric diagnostic interview examination (CPT code 90801)
➠ end-state renal disease–related services (HCPCS codes G0308, G0309, G0311, G0314, G0315, G0317, and G0318)
➠ Individual Medical Nutrition Therapy (HCPCS codes G0270, 97802, and 97803).

The secretary of HHS also has the independent legislative authority to add services as he or she deems appropriate for Medicare reimbursement.

Claims for Medicare reimbursement for telemedicine services are submitted with the telehealth modifier "GT" which indicates that the service was delivered using a live-interactive telecommunications system. Store-and-forward services in Alaska and Hawaii use a "GQ" modifier.

Although Medicare reimbursement for telemedicine was expanded in the 106th Congress and CMS has an annual process for expanding reimbursement, it still lags behind the private sector and lacks the innovation in telemedicine reimbursement present in many state Medicaid programs. Medicare does not reimburse for telemedicine services delivered to patients located in urban areas; however, many urban patients have significant barriers to accessing quality healthcare delivered by the most appropriate healthcare provider in a timely fashion. For example, easy access to linguistically and culturally competent healthcare providers may be lacking for urban patients. This gap may be easily bridged with live-interactive telehealth.

Over 5 years have passed since the Medicare telemedicine reimbursement expansion of October 1, 2001. While the federal Congressional Budget Office (CBO) predicted that this expansion would cost taxpayers $150 million over 5 years, it actually cost less than $3 million. Given the past 6 years of evidence demonstrating that telemedicine reimbursement does not necessarily lead to overutilization, further expansion of Medicare reimbursement for telemedicine in the future is expected.

Medicaid/SCHIP

According to the CMS, states are using telemedicine technologies for reasons including "increased cost efficiency, reduced transportation expenses, improved patient access to specialists and mental health providers, improved quality of care, and better communication among providers" [1]. While this is a dynamic area, at the present time over half the states in the United States have some reimbursement regulations for telehealth services and 23 states now have specific Medicaid regulations that provide for reimbursement for telemedicine services. Most of the states that reimburse for telemedicine through Medicaid and SCHIP recognize physician consultations (medical and mental health) when they are furnished using live-interactive telemedicine. Payment is usually on a fee-for-service basis and is the same as the reimbursement for covered services furnished for a traditional in-person visit. Reimbursement is sometimes made at both ends (hub and spoke sites) and most states use consultative CPT codes with the modifier "TM" to identify telemedicine services, although a variety of different modifiers are in use [1].

Most state legislation mandating reimbursement for telemedicine services for Medicaid beneficiaries provides for care delivered via telemedicine if the care is a covered benefit when provided in person; however, various reimbursement restrictions exist. Medicaid in Nebraska covers services as long as comparable services are not available to the patient within a 30-mile radius of his or her home. Utah Medicaid is very specific in the type of provider (e.g., psychiatrist, psychologist, social workers, psychiatric registered nurse, and certified marriage and family therapists) eligible for reimbursement. The California Medicaid program Medi-Cal requires documentation of the reason for using telemedicine [2]. The list of reasons includes

⮞ geographic barriers
⮞ local provider unavailable
⮞ local provider wait time unacceptable
⮞ local provider unwilling to accept Medi-Cal
⮞ local provider unable to address lingual or cultural needs of the patient
⮞ transportation unavailable
⮞ time off work creates personal or professional hardship.

Store-and-forward telemedicine services, such as store-and-forward teledermatology, are recognized in medical assistance programs in several states including South Dakota, Minnesota, Texas, and California. Teledermatology is sometimes singled out as uniquely appropriate for store-and-forward reimbursement, such as the decision in California to add store-and-forward teledermatology and teleophthamology to the list of consultative services that are reimbursed by Medi-Cal (California Medicaid) as of mid-2006.

Private payer reimbursement

In many states private payers have taken the lead on telemedicine reimbursement, including reimbursement for teledermatology. In 2002, the ATA and AMD Telemedicine contacted 72 active telemedicine programs and asked about payment received from private payers. More than half of the programs contacted were receiving reimbursement from private payers. This limited sampling found over 100 private payers that reimbursed for telemedicine services in at least 25 states. Today, this number is up to nearly 150, including Blue Cross/Blue Shield plans who reimburse for telemedicine services in at least 21 states [3].

Some states have taken steps to mandate private payer reimbursement for telemedicine services. These states have typically enacted legislation that prevents exclusion of coverage if the service is provided via telemedicine. Examples follow:

⮞ Louisiana SB 773 (1995)
⮞ California SB 1665 (1996)
⮞ Oklahoma SB 48 (1997)

- Texas HB 2033 (1997)
- Kentucky HB 177 (2000)
- Colorado (in rural areas) (2001).

Established telemedicine programs across the country have been successful in obtaining private payer reimbursement for live-interactive telemedicine by treating the services as usual and customary, sending a letter to the private payer describing the intent to provide telemedicine services, notifying the payer about future claim submittals, and asking if special modifiers are required. The payer is simply asked to respond with any comments or questions. This procedure has been used in multiple states with a variety of private payers with positive results. In most instances, private payers either do not issue a response or they respond stating that special coding is not required. Customary billing procedures are adhered to and the claims are processed and paid.

Rural and frontier areas are more likely to have private payers who reimburse for live-interactive telemedicine. For example, Marquette General Health System, in the upper peninsula of Michigan, reports that "95% of telemedicine services provided in our region are reimbursable by third-party payers" [4].

Private payer reimbursement for store-and-forward teledermatology exists in California where Blue Cross Commercial, Blue Cross State Sponsored Programs, and California Public Employees' Retirement System (CALPERS) all reimburse for store-and-forward teledermatology consults. Partners Health System in Boston also receives reimbursement from BC/BS for store-and-forward follow-up visits for patients with acne as part of a clinical trial. Given the lack of access to dermatology across the United States, increased examples of private payer reimbursement for store-and-forward teledermatology are expected.

"Closed" or vertically integrated healthcare systems

Reimbursement schema for teledermatology services are less prevalent in so-called closed or vertically integrated healthcare systems such as correctional healthcare, the VA healthcare system, and DOD's care of active duty military personnel. In these systems access to care rather than revenue generation via reimbursement is often the driving force. Additionally, cost avoidance through contracted dermatology care or subsidized "out of system" care is an economic consideration. That is not to say that if Medicare billing rules change, teledermatology will not be a source of revenue in these settings. Nonetheless, the current incentives in these systems foster and support the development of both live-interactive and store-and-forward teledermatology programs. Many veterans live in rural, underserved areas and access the VA healthcare system via remote Community Based Outpatient Clinics that mainly deliver primary medical care and busy dermatologists in the DOD system can use teledermatology to triage their case loads and target their in-person care where it is most urgently needed. Both LI and S/F teledermatology can be used in these settings. It is not uncommon to see innovations in teledermatology from these closed systems derived from the need to provide specialty care to sites that are remote from the centralized medical centers and hospitals.

Reimbursement for the uninsured through grants

National, state, and local health foundations provide reimbursement for the uninsured via telehealth. The federal Office for the Advancement of Telehealth (OAT) has long provided similar support for uninsured patients through their grants and contracting programs. Because teledermatology is frequently used to access remote, underserved patient populations, health foundations may be interested in supporting this improved access. The Missouri Foundation for Health, for example, provides reimbursement through a grant for patients seen through the Missouri Telehealth Network if no other source of funding is available.

Contracts supporting reimbursement

A variety of contractual arrangements exist for teledermatology services in both the public and private sectors. These contracts may be between large employers and dermatology provider groups, between local/state governments and teledermatology service providers, or between academic dermatology departments and foreign countries. One example is a contract for teledermatology services from the University of Miami for dermatological care of active duty military secondary to a shortage of military dermatologists due to deployment. As teledermatology expands, the growth of fee-for-service or per capitation contractual arrangements is expected.

Correctional healthcare contracts in which the dermatologists share in the financial risk are also conducive to teledermatology. Transportation costs for prisoners tend to be very high and use of telemedicine technologies in areas where quality has been demonstrated, such as teledermatology, is commonsensical. In fact, teledermatology has been used successfully for the management of prisoners in many states. The Arizona Telemedicine Program [5] has been caring for prisoners from four locations using telemedicine since 1997. Currently, over 80% of their specialty visits, including dermatology, for prisoners are conducted via telehealth and millions of dollars have been saved.

Emerging reimbursement models

A multitude of new business and reimbursement models, discussed in the previous chapter, are emerging. Patients are increasingly willing to pay out of pocket for access and convenience. There is a current move toward transparency in both the cost of and quality of healthcare services. As the technology evolves and patients are increasingly able to obtain high-quality digital photos of their own skin conditions or that of their family members or friends, direct patient to dermatologist interaction at the convenience of both is easy to imagine. How this type of care will be reimbursed and by whom remains to be seen.

REFERENCES

[1] CMS web site. Available at http://www.cms.hhs.gov/default.asp? Last accessed on April 15, 2007.
[2] The California Telemedicine and eHealth Center (CTEC) http://www.ctecon line.org/pdf/Telemedicine%20Reimbursement%20Handbook%20FINAL.pdf Last accessed on April 15, 2007.
[3] AMD-ATA Private Payer Survey. Available at http://www.amdtelemedicine.com/ private_payer/about_survey.html Last accessed on April 15, 2007.
[4] Marquette General Hospital web site. Available at http://www.mgh.org/. Last accessed on April 15, 2007.
[5] Arizona Telemedicine Program. Available at http://www.telemedicine.arizona. edu/. Last accessed on April 15, 2007.

8 Getting started*

Joseph Tracy, Karen E. Edison, and Hon S. Pak

If you are interested in developing a teledermatology program, this chapter is for you. There are a multitude of variables that need to be considered in developing a teledermatology practice. These variables include understanding the types of teledermatology modalities available, understanding how teledermatology fits your organization, being knowledgeable about the legal and regulatory issues impacting the program, being familiar with your reimbursement landscape, and most importantly understanding the intrinsic and extrinsic reasons and rewards for wanting to offer the teledermatology.

This chapter assumes that the reader has read the chapters describing the rationale for teledermatology, potential business models available, and how reimbursement for those services is obtained. This chapter concentrates on other issues that need to be considered before starting a teledermatology program. We also describe ways to implement and provide teledermatology services in three ways – via live-interactive video (LIV), store-and-forward (S/F), and a hybrid method using both LIV and S/F technologies.

The reader should note that starting any telehealth project is a time-consuming process. Ideally, one should allow a 6-month window of time to devote to researching, planning, and implementing a teledermatology program. Disciplined planning will increase your chance of being successful.

For private practice dermatologists, we have prepared an abridged version of this chapter in an effort to make it more relevant for solo or small practice dermatologists (see Appendix H, this book).

Do your homework (step 1)

The first step is to ascertain the degree to which a telehealth program either falls within the existing scope of the practice or how the development of the

---

* Adapted from the Teledermatology Technical Assistance Document written by the same authors posted on the OAT web site.

teledermatology service might benefit the practice's mission. Much of the consideration depends on the dermatologist's practice (e.g., general dermatology, MOHS, pediatric, etc.) and the practice setting (e.g., solo or group). Consideration must also be given to whether or not the program will be developed within the confines of a well-established practice or whether it will be used to help jumpstart a developing practice.

In addition, a telehealth plan for the practice must be developed. This requires several initial tasks:

1. Review the literature and the web to get a full understanding and appreciation for what existing organizations are doing in teledermatology. Chapter 3 of this book provides an excellent review on current utilization of teledermatology. Other sources of information can be found by visiting several of the following web sites (last accessed on May 4, 2007):

   a) American Telemedicine Association – www.americantelemed.org
   b) Association of Telemedicine Service Providers – www.atsp.org
   c) Center for Telehealth and eHealth Law – www.ctel.org
   d) Federal Office for the Advancement of Telehealth – http://tele-health.hrsa.gov/
   e) Telemedicine Information Exchange – http://tie.telemed.org/
   f) A Guide to Getting Started in Telemedicine – http://telehealth.muhealth.org/geninfo/TAD.html
   g) American Academy of Dermatology: Teledermatology Guideline – http://www.aad.org/professionals/policies/Policies.htm (select telemedicine).
   h) National Telehealth Law Center – www.telehealthlawcenter.org

Planning the program to meet the needs of the target population (step 2)

Whether one is looking to create a live-interactive or S/F teledermatology program, it is important to understand the geographic areas and the demographics of the population intended to be served. In this process the reader should do the following:

1. Assess the needs/demand for dermatology services in the target area via existing databases (e.g., state listing of specialists) and interviews with primary care providers. Obtain answers to the following questions:

   a) Are there dermatologists in the target area (within the same or neighboring county)?
   b) Where do patients in the target area currently go to receive dermatology services?
   c) If dermatology services were available via telemedicine would they be of benefit to the provider?
   d) How often would the provider use the service?

2. Assess the current referral relationship between the target area primary care physicians (PCP) and the dermatologist(s), if any, operating in the area by obtaining answers to such questions as:
   a) Is the current dermatology referral relationship and service positive, or is the relationship poor?
   If the relationship is poor:
   1. Is the PCP seeking alternatives because the dermatologist they have used in the past is booked beyond his/her capacity or is not providing a valued service?
   2. Is the PCP looking for an alternative because the dermatologist they have used in the past has decided to accept only paying patients?
   3. Is the current relationship coming to an end as a result of retirement, relocation, or some other reason?
3. Consider the existing relationships between the target area's providers (e.g., physicians, hospitals, health department, etc.) and the short-term and long-term impact of implementing of telehealth in that area. In this process it is likely that potential partners will be identified (unless they sought the dermatology service on their own). However, in some cases one may also find that the providers in any given area do not want to work with their local dermatologist or their institution for a variety of reasons (e.g., poor service, lack of confidence in the provider).
4. Assess the population of people necessary to support a dermatologist in the target area by contacting local health agencies, university-based health management programs, or through health planning publications. The ability to recruit a dermatologist to an area insufficient in population to support such a provider will be difficult if not impossible. Teledermatology access may fill that gap.
5. In addition to understanding the needs and demands of the population to be served, many questions like the following need to be answered:
   a) Why should the practice use telemedicine?
   b) If it is an established practice, "Does the practice have the capacity to handle additional patients?"
   c) "If the practice doesn't provide a telemedicine service, will a competitor?"
   d) If a new practice, "Can telemedicine expand the reach of the practice, help to build relationships with other providers, and attract patients into the practice at a faster pace than might otherwise be possible without the technology?"
   e) If a pediatric dermatology practice, "How can telemedicine be used to expand the service to other geographic areas that will provide the population base necessary to support the practice?"
   f) If a Cutaneous Micrographic (Moh's) Surgery practice, "Will telemedicine provide the ability to see post-op wound checks in a more efficient patient-centered manner so that more new cases can be

seen in person? Or will teledermatology increase the referral to your Moh's practice?"

6. Based on the literature review (see Chapter 4) and the need/demand analysis, develop a conservative budget to illustrate what the program might cost. Both short- and long-term sustainability issues should be considered.

7. Research the availability of third-party funding for the service (grants, contracts). Depending upon the state in which that practice is located, the telemedicine administrator for the practice needs to lay the groundwork with third-party payers for the purposes of reimbursement for services delivered via telemedicine. It will be easier to educate third-party payers before beginning the program to assure that they understand what teledermatology is and how it will be used. Even if legislation is in place that requires them to pay, they can be resistant if they do not understand telehealth.

8. Develop an executive summary and more detailed report based on the information gathered in the first two steps. Depending upon the type of practice – group, multispecialty group, academic practice, and the like – provide the executive summary and report to other decision makers and ask for support. Without a high level of commitment from all the key stakeholders, the program will not evolve and become an accepted component of the practice.

Implementation (step 3)

Once the decision has been made to proceed, it is imperative to follow the steps below. For smaller clinics or organizations whose resources may be limited, one may consider partnering or consulting with an organization/ vendor, which can provide this service.

1. Appoint or hire the following individuals whose duties will be to make the program work:
   a) program administrator
   b) clinical coordinator

2. Contact a few established teledermatology programs that are similar to the one being proposed and arrange for one or more site visits. A site visit, if well planned, will provide a wealth of information regarding clinic logistics, policies, and protocols.

3. Promote the concept to other physicians in the practice along with the nurses, other clinical providers, and administration. It is important to get these individuals involved from the beginning to avoid any uphill battles later on.

4. Consider holding a stakeholder's meeting to discuss telehealth with the potential partners and originating site community. This may include individuals from the city/town council, business and industry leaders, school board members, and of course members engaged in the delivery

of healthcare services. Such a meeting gives the telehealth providers a chance to discover concerns, fears, support, and desires on the part of the local community. The meeting should include a general overview of teledermatology and how it works to meet patient needs. In this first meeting the presenter should recommend that the community create an advisory group to assess and support the telehealth concept. It may also include discussions on how to make competing institutions partners in telehealth. The presenter should also address costs, benefits, and barriers during this meeting.

5. Consider hosting a separate "due diligence" meeting with many healthcare providers to assure them that telehealth is being used in the community to provide dermatology services that do not exist and not as a tool to drain patients from the area. Provide as much information to the originating site providers as possible in order to give them some idea of what they can expect. In this meeting, the following items should be included:

a) The dermatologist must attend. Healthcare providers prefer to know the specialists to whom they refer their patients. Have the dermatologist explain how he or she will communicate back with the referring providers regarding their patients. This may be via written documentation that is faxed, sent via secure email, or via the traditional dictated letter. Inform them that such a response will be clear and timely. Additionally, offer the originating site providers an easy communication channel for asking questions of the dermatologists. If objections are raised regarding the communication methods, then ask the providers how they would like to receive feedback on the patients they will refer.

b) Convey to the originating site providers that as news gets out into the originating site community about this service, patients will begin to refer themselves. Additionally, let the dermatologists at the distant site know that they need to decide if they will accept direct patient referrals, and if they do accept them, how they will remotely manage patients with complicated conditions. Remember that accepting direct referrals without prior approval of some insurance companies could create a complicated reimbursement environment. Convey to the referring providers how the dermatologists would prefer to handle telemedicine cases. There are three ways this is typically done:

- The dermatologist can assume responsibility for the patient's initial and follow-up care.
- The dermatologist can partner with the patient's primary care provider and comanage the patient.
- The dermatologist may choose to provide only consultative recommendations to the primary care provider for the patient's management.

In short, the dermatologists will need to decide which method they would prefer to use or whether they will make the determination on a case-by-case basis. It should be noted that dermatologists using only S/F technology will customarily be serving in a purely consultative role.

a) Request that the originating site providers become part of a directory that will list everyone in the community capable of providing surgical and other procedural expertise (e.g., skin biopsy, simple excisions, cryosurgery, and intralesional injections). This way the patient can remain local when such expertise is needed. This is another indication that telemedicine will help healthcare service remain in the underserved area. Please note that if this type of procedural expertise is not available, the patient may need to travel out of the local community for such services.

b) Offer the referring providers the opportunity to spend time with the dermatologists in their clinics learning basic procedural techniques. In this way, full-service modern dermatology care may be provided in the underserved areas. Additionally, offer the staff of the referring providers (e.g., LPNs, RNs) an opportunity to also spend time with the dermatologists and their staff for the purpose of learning the procedural techniques and how the dermatologists utilize the skills of their staff during patient encounters.

6. Clearly define the measurable goals/objectives for the teledermatology service. Those objectives should have clear timelines and the name of the individual responsible for the objective.

7. Refine the estimated costs to the practice and the partner sites. Remember antikickback laws will prevent your practice from funding equipment and network connections to your partner sites.

8. Design a method for data collection and analysis so that a financial "look back" can be provided on a periodic basis so that the program can make adjustments, if necessary.

9. Develop a telehealth agreement with the designated site. This agreement should define the responsibilities of each party including staffing, costs, technical support, reporting, and the like. In this process the reader should have gathered sample agreements from other telehealth programs. They should be used as the basis for the agreements that the reader will draft. AN AGREEMENT MUST BE FINALIZED WITH EACH SITE BEFORE MOVING TO THE OPERATIONAL STAGE. Otherwise, false expectations and misunderstandings may arise regarding which party is responsible for providing services, staffing, and equipment for the teledermatology service.

Perform a technical analysis

The practice will need to consult with both telecommunications and information technology experts in the design and development of the technical infrastructure. Depending on the size of the practice these individuals may already be part of the practice. If not, hiring experts would be advisable. Those embarking on a teledermatology program should begin their technical analysis by

1. identifying teledermatology equipment used by other successful programs;
2. identifying transmission mechanisms used by other successful programs;
3. reviewing the American Telemedicine Association's Teledermatology Special Interest Group web site – http://www.americantelemed.org/ICOT/icot.htm (last accessed on May 4, 2007). This link has a wealth of information regarding both live-interactive and S/F teledermatology.
4. *being sure to allow the teledermatologists to test and participate in the final selection of the equipment*.

Technical considerations for LIV, S/F, and hybrid teledermatology

1. Determine how ongoing maintenance of equipment will be provided. This includes a decision to buy spare equipment or extended service contracts. It may be less expensive to buy spare devices when the equipment has a warranty of 2–3 years. That way, the spare can be placed in the field while the broken equipment is repaired under its warranty period.
2. Determine network connectivity options and associated costs. This means exploring all the types of telecommunication services that may be available in the target area (e.g., ISDN, xDSL, T1, IP). If considering S/F as the modality, plain old telephone service (POTS) or cable *may* suffice.
3. Determine who will be responsible for network management from point to point – the distant site, originating site, the telecommunications company, or some third party.
4. Train the telehealth technical staff on proper room design. This includes understanding proper lighting (for videoconferencing and S/F), sound, and video placement for optimal telehealth presentations. For S/F teledermatology it should also involve training the user on the techniques needed to take and transmit digital images of the patient. A couple considerations include:
   a) Lighting should be adequate enough to identify the primary lesions and their characteristics.
   b) A medium nonreflectant blue cloth or blue screen background should be used so that there is continuity in the images taken. The color should be similar to that used for blue screens in Hollywood.
   c) Clothing and jewelry must be removed sufficiently to get adequate viewing.

    d) Use chaperones as needed to assist the patient.

    e) For S/F or hybrid teledermatology, use of an imaging protocol is highly recommended (see Appendix D, this book).

5. Develop agreements to determine what happens when equipment is stolen or damaged.

6. Consider the development of procedures and policy for equipment utilization and network connectivity. It should include the following:

    a) Indicate how teledermatology connections between sites are to be scheduled and which site places the call (e.g., set block of time each week, ad hoc, scheduled into an existing clinic, distant site makes the call) and

    b) indicate how each piece of equipment works and how it interfaces with the video system or S/F system).

7. Develop a frequently asked questions (FAQ) sheet that will help reduce the stress imposed by the Health Insurance Portability and Accountability Act (HIPAA). This should be done in conjunction with the distant site's privacy and security staff.

8. Create an inventory tracking system for all equipment.

Operational

Steps 1–3 in this chapter are likely to take 6 or more months before the operational stage is entered. The timelines below start only after steps 1–3 are completed. Please remember not to embark on an operational plan until a formal telehealth agreement is in place with the originating site.

Start-up – the first 30 days

If the teledermatology program has an emphasis on providing services in rural areas, the IT staff should be aware of and take advantage of the FCC's Universal Service Mechanism for Health Care. This mechanism provides discounts on broadband telecommunication services to certain rural healthcare facilities. Many times the Universal Service Mechanism makes the difference between affording vs not affording a connection to a rural telemedicine site. If applicable, Universal Service Fund applications should be filed with the Rural Health Care Division (RHCD) of the Universal Service Administration Corporation. While this step can happen quickly, do not order the telecommunications service until the 28-day waiting period required by the RHCD has expired as otherwise the service will not qualify for Universal Service funding. Soliciting bids or comparison-shopping needs to be done to ensure best pricing of equipment and telecommunication services. Blind bidding can produce a large variation in pricing and save a great deal of money. Locating existing bids within the institution for videoconferencing equipment, cameras, and the like, may also save time in the purchasing process.

1. Conduct additional site visits for finalizing the technical placement of all equipment.
2. Determine the general layout of the room and what changes (lighting, sound, wall color), if any, need to be made. The telehealth agreement with the site should specify which party is responsible for any room modifications and wire pulls.
3. Hold administrative and clinical meetings to discuss the logistics of scheduling, billing, reimbursement, evaluation, consent, and other administrative issues related to the program.
4. Observe in detail how in-person clinics function and detail how tele-health will best fit into that environment. Provide the staff at the underserved site with information that details the ideal real-time or S/F encounter.

The 31–60-day start-up window

1. Continue working on all of the logistical issues related to scheduling, billing, and so on.
2. Order telecommunications services AFTER THE RHCD 28-DAY WINDOW CLOSES (if filing RHCD paperwork was applicable).
3. Order all equipment.
4. Room remodeling, if needed, should begin around day 31. This includes any necessary cabinetry, wall mounts, painting, and the like, to be completed by the 60th day.
5. Develop or locate existing evaluation tools to pilot in the next step. Each telehealth program will need to determine if the evaluation tools need to be academic (e.g., comparing dermatology diagnoses with telemedicine vs traditional in-person care), financial (e.g., cost/bene-fit), or simply capture general utilization (e.g., patient origin, number of studies by diagnosis code, etc.) data.

The 61–90-day start-up window

1. Install equipment.
2. Configure and connect network devices.
3. Test all equipment and network connections thoroughly for quality of service and security.
4. Begin scheduling hands-on training sessions for the staff in the target community (physicians, nurses, other clinical staff and administrative staff). This includes training on hardware, software, and perhaps traveling to the distant site (dermatologist site) to do some clinical and technical training with the dermatologist and his or her staff. See Appendix C for training consult managers using S/F technologies.
5. Finalize the logistics of scheduling, billing, medical record keeping, medical record sharing, and the like.

6. Conduct mock cases to determine the smoothness of the process and to make refinements as necessary. This process should go from the referral process to the evaluation forms (if used) completed at the end of an encounter.

The 91st day – time for patient care

1. Begin caring for patients based on the groundwork laid during the first 90 days.
2. Refinements and adjustments to the program can be made at this point.
3. Begin collecting data as per the evaluation plan developed earlier.

Sustainment

Even after extensive planning, implementation, and training, you will need a team to provide close follow-up for the next several months to ensure that no new issues (business vs technical) arise which may lead to quick disuse. In fact most of the problems encountered relate not to the technical aspect but rather human factors and other nontelemedicine issues. The bottom line is that the earlier you intervene, the higher the chance of success. You must also establish a quality control program which ensures that the quality of the clinical information and the images are adequate and that there is a mechanism set up to ensure that issues are addressed appropriately and in a timely fashion, especially in the early stages. To this extent, you must have a sustainable (financially) program and a team that will provide timely customer support. Last, you must coordinate with each referring facility to ensure that the metrics are being collected appropriately and that a reporting mechanism is in place.

Lessons learned from the field

1. *Dermatologists will experience a learning curve of an unknown time*: Confidence levels correlate with diagnostic accuracy. New teledermatologists may want to see patients in person and via teledermatology for an initial period of time until they become comfortable with their ability to render quality dermatological care.
2. *Originating site healthcare providers will also experience a learning curve of an unknown time*: It takes time for the originating site healthcare providers, presenters, and image technicians to learn how to deliver teledermatology services. Each originating site will take varying amounts of time depending upon the amount of support and time given to the teledermatology service.
3. *Teledermatology is less difficult to implement if referral relationships with primary care providers in the community are already established*: However, this may not be the case, because communities with the

greatest need for teledermatology typically lack easy access to dermatological services.

4. *Teledermatology services will have a greater chance of success if the dermatologists are willing to drive to the community, meet with the medical staff, and perhaps give a dermatology lecture from time to time*: As in standard referral relationships, telehealth referral relationships are based on human connections and excellent service rendered over the long term.

5. *Primary care providers need to know to whom they are referring their patients*: If in-person communications or visits are not possible, schedule a videoconference for the dermatologists to meet and greet the originating site physicians. Interactive educational programs via the network can also serve to introduce the dermatologists to the referring providers.

6. *The dermatologist should discuss with the originating site medical staff what level of service they are prepared to render*: They may act as a consultant, as a comanager, and sometimes as a direct caregiver for the patients. This of course depends on the clinical diagnosis and treatment plan. Additionally, ask the primary care providers to comment on what level of service they are expecting when they write a request for consultation via the teledermatology service.

7. *Keeping the originating site healthcare workers adept at using the equipment is an ongoing challenge*: As with any telehealth service, teledermatology works best when clinics are frequently held. Even in the best of circumstances, personnel will come and go and take their expertise with them. Thus, be prepared for retraining camera users and image photographers in all locations.

8. *Use standard operating procedures and protocols for teledermatology encounters*: A standard protocol for patient presentation (LIV and hybrid), for gathering a patient history (LIV, S/F, and hybrid), and for patient imaging (S/F, LIV, and hybrid) should be used.

9. *Always take multiple images of the patient (S/F and hybrid).*

10. *Never take a picture at less than 6–12 in. (will vary with digital camera) from the patient (S/F and hybrid).*

11. *Consider turning off the flash when photographing the scalp, particularly in a patient with dark-colored hair (S/F and hybrid)*: The flash will wash out the image of the underlying scalp if it is used in this case.

12. *If images need to be retaken at the request of the dermatologist ensure that the referring sites do not see this as an insult to their skills and abilities*: Use the retake session as a learning opportunity to improve on the process.

Conclusion

If a teledermatology program is implemented correctly in the appropriate setting, it can make a significant difference in improving access to and quality of care while reducing or containing cost. Careful attention to the elements of implementation described in this chapter will greatly increase opportunities for success. Deciding on whether to start a teledermatology program requires that you understand your personal and organizational values and whether it makes both clinical and financial sense. Following the steps outlined in this chapter and relying on the experience of others will assist you to determine if teledermatology is right for you and help you learn how to go about setting up a teledermatology program.

9 Ethical implications in the use of telehealth and teledermatology

David A. Fleming

There's no going back. We are headed for a future where healthcare will be dominated by information and communication technologies, and like it or not we must learn how to adapt and use it skillfully and effectively for the good of our patients. In so many ways, healthcare is improved by techno-logical innovations that allow us to effectively diagnose and treat illness and relieve suffering. However, as technology evolves and as the skills necessary to use that technology become increasingly difficult and selective to attain, so grows the risk that healthcare will become *technology* centric rather than *patient* centric.

Multiple forms of informational technology are rapidly being developed and deployed. Electronic medical records, telephone intervention and triage centers, email diagnosis and prescribing, transmission of medical images, remote monitoring, and videoconferencing are all inundating the health-care field. For healthcare providers to remain focused on their primary goal, a studied and balanced approach must be taken that will allow the intro-duction of innovative interventions without losing sight of the patient as having unique needs, recognizing that there is potential for harm and abuse, and that "one size does not fit all" in the application of new forms of treat-ment and technology. Stanberry argues that telehealth presents us with unique and ethically appropriate opportunities for both the patient and the clinician when it is implemented in direct response to clear clinical needs, but warns against excessive reliance upon technology to the detriment of traditional provider-patient relationships and cautions against complacen-cy regarding the risks and responsibilities that distant medical intervention, consultation, and diagnosis carry [1].

There is no reason why the efficiencies of information and communi-cation technology should not allow us to reconnect with the reason we became physicians in the first place – to selflessly use our skills and knowledge to make a difference in the lives of and improve the welfare of others. The use of any technology in healthcare should not become a barrier to prudent clinical judgment, undermine the healing relationship, or be a means in to itself. In short, telehealth, like any evolving healthcare technology, should be used in such a way that will allow us to function optimally as healthcare professionals, and to connect with (rather than detract from) our own humanity, as well as that of our patients.

In this chapter we discuss the ethical implications in the use of tele-health – more specifically how these ethical concerns apply to the unique application of both live-interactive and store-and-forward teledermatology. Ethical concerns in the use of telehealth have been identified [2–5] but will be explored in more detail. The ethical implications of telehealth go well beyond the expectation to respect patient autonomy, from which springs providers' obligations to ensuring informed consent, privacy, and confidentiality. The ethical ambivalence of telehealth relates to the uniquely positive impact that telehealth can have on the patient, the provider, and clinical outcomes as well as the potential for harm and abuse that may ensue. Arguably, one of the most contentious concerns in the field today is the potential impact that "virtual care" or "distance care" has on the healing relationship that traditionally forms between patients and their providers. The loss of touch, the potential for depersonalization, and the danger of virtual visits "replacing" actual visits in the interest of cost savings and time efficiency are palpable concerns. In addition, the challenges of providing reasonable access to unevenly deployed services and the possibility of inequity is very real when considering the benefits that can be derived from telehealth and teledermatology. There is also the potential that as healthcare technology moves into the home (such as teledermatology from the home computer), it may impose a burden on sick and vulnerable patients who do not understand the technology or feel it may be intrusive. Finally, the question of legitimacy of purpose and the potential for exploitation is a very clear and present ethical concern that cannot be avoided in today's market-driven medical environment.

Autonomy: Consent, privacy, and confidentiality

Medical tradition is grounded by the healing relationship, which is based on the trust of one who is ill (the patient) shared with another (the physician) who has the nonproprietary skill and knowledge to heal, and commits herself to doing so by taking an oath. Traditionally there has also been a normative acceptance of patient rights and the physician's *prima facie* obligation (which is to say, duties that always apply unless other overriding obligations exist) to respect and advocate for those rights. The physician must also consider other interests, such as those of the family, the health-care organization, and society, when making clinical judgments and utilizing resources, but for the treating physician these accessory interests remain ethically subsidiary to those of the patient.

The principle of respect for patient autonomy requires that the clinician do all he or she reasonably can to respect the patient's right to make an informed decision pertaining to actions the clinician may or may not take in his or her behalf and to have personal information protected. It also requires physicians to keep encounters with patients private, whether in person (actual) or electronic (virtual), unless the patient requests or gives permission for personal information to be shared. One ethical concern that has surfaced with the advent of expanding means of communicating electronically and at distances is that confidentiality may become less important or more difficult to enforce. Breaking confidentiality can be classified as breaches of security or inappropriate disclosure of individual patient information to unauthorized persons. Such inadvertent or inappropriate disclosure can be both visual and auditory, such as the unauthorized viewing or hearing of videoconferenced interactions with patients, or viewing photos of skin lesions or other electronic medical records that have been received from another provider or retrieved from an otherwise protected database. Unauthorized access or use of any form of patient information is unethical and typically not in compliance with organizational regulatory policies regarding privacy.

In a report of Internet users seeking health information on the web, personal privacy was ranked as the most important concern [6]. Confidential information should be protected whenever transmitted, stored, received, or otherwise disposed of to ensure that patient confidentiality is respected and personal identifiable information protected. Unauthorized, and often quite innocent, disclosure or viewing may occur with both live-interactive and store-and-forward interactions, thus technological, as well as personal, safeguards are necessary to keep all electronic interactions private and inaccessible to those who are unauthorized [7].

The requirement of informed consent is also an important ethical consideration for telehealth. Unfortunately, however, there seems to be less diligence in making sure that patients are well informed and provide appropriate consent prior to photo or video interventions compared to other, more traditional, forms of clinical intervention [8]. The use of telehealth technology, whether by videoconferencing or store-and-forward, is still a clinical intervention and has the potential to both positively and negatively impact the health and welfare of the patient. It should never be presumed, therefore, that others can sit in on discussion or that information, such as photos of skin lesions and personal historical information, can be shared unless authorized by the patient or their surrogate.

Clinical interactions with patients occur on a continuum over time and likewise consent should continuously be sought if others are going to be present during telehealth interactions and if information, such as photos, is to be shared with colleagues in order to optimize clinical decisions or for educational purposes. If patients are not effectively informed and consented prior to telehealth interventions, then the dignity, autonomy, and well-being of patients cannot truly be protected. Informed consent, a requirement of professional respect for the patient, should be an ongoing and open-ended process incorporated into any clinical intervention, whether face to face or electronic, either of which may be at risk for inadvertent or unwanted disclosure.

Provider-patient relationships

The ethical and legal principles that apply to conventional face-to-face provider-patient relationships are equally valid for both videoconferencing and store-and-forward telehealth interactions [9]. This means that the use of telehealth must not adversely affect the mutual relationship of trust and respect shared by the patient and provider, the independent judgment of the provider, or the autonomous decision making for the patient.

But, is there a danger that telehealth and other forms of information technology will ultimately replace the patient as the ultimate goal of treatment? A tragic and ironic fallacy would be if the patient were to be marginalized as the "data source" for transmitting information to the physician while technology itself becomes the goal and purpose of the clinical moment. Many argue that physical proximity is still important to securing the common links and reciprocal connections important to this trust relationship and that telehealth should function as an adjunct to, not a replacement of, the traditional physical encounter that frames the clinical moment [10–12]. Telehealth, as with any healthcare technology, should be utilized as yet one more tool to improve the care and treatment of patients but not replace the face-to-face relationship that remains crucial to healing.

Finland, having developed a robust nationwide telehealth network, recognizes the potential deleterious impact that telehealth may have on the healing relationship. In 1997 the Finnish Medical Association developed ethical guidelines for the use of telemedicine, which states that "Preferably all patients seeking medical advice should see a doctor in a face to face consultation, and telemedicine should be restricted to situations in which a doctor can not be physically present within acceptable time" [13]. It is argued that telemedicine should be restricted to situations in which a patient cannot physically see a provider within an acceptable period of time, the major application being consultation by the patient's treating physician or at the request of the patient. For consultation, of course, it is infrequent that the patient and physician know each other prior to the clinic visit, and it is therefore important that the patient's referring physician know and trust the telehealth specialist to whom the patient is being referred if telehealth is the preferred or only realistic option for the patient.

The impact of the physician's physical presence and touch on the patient-physician relationship and the perception of patients as a result of face-to-face interactions have been demonstrated and cannot be discounted [14]. A recent study examining the attitudes of attending physicians and residents regarding the use of telehealth in training found that the potential impact of using telehealth on the physician-patient relationship was an important concern [15]. Though 90% of resident and attending physicians felt telehealth would improve patient care, only 37% felt it would have a positive impact on relationships with patients and 75% were uncomfortable assessing new patients by telehealth. Most physicians (79%) were also uncomfortable having difficult discussions with patients via telehealth, such as breaking bad news, and the vast majority were not comfortable making difficult diagnosis and treatment decisions without the patient being physically present (95%). This survey, however, was of physicians with no prior telehealth experience. Users of telehealth technology uniformly have more positive impressions.

For patients telehealth is often favored over face-to-face visits. An analysis of 38 telehealth studies revealed that, in general, both patients and providers were satisfied with care when telehealth technology was used. In fact, doctor-patient communication via telehealth was often favored over face-to-face communication by both providers and patients, at the same time enabling cost savings, such as decreased utilization of skilled nursing visits and a decrease in the number of repeat hospitalizations for certain groups of patients [16]. Other studies, however, emphasize that telehealth technology should be used as an adjunct to the care and treatment provided to patients. Even when providers had positive perceptions of telehealth, they emphasized that it was an additional tool and not a substitute for actual visits [17].

Justice, access, and equity

Equity springs from social justice and the notion of fair distribution of social goods, such as healthcare, is a widely accepted normative principle by which we function as healthcare professionals. Yet, a growing number of Americans, presently 46.6 million, do not have adequate access to healthcare [18]. Those without access live in both urban and rural areas and tend to be isolated from providers due to physical as well as economic barriers, including lack of healthcare benefits, geography, and immobility. Disparities in healthcare access also tend to run along ethnic and racial differences lines in parallel to poverty [19]. Finding ways to provide healthcare for those isolated, without access, and unfairly made vulnerable to illness and premature death is an ethical imperative for society.

One of the most challenging problems confronting healthcare today is the uneven distribution and relative shortage of providers in rural areas [20]. Despite concerted efforts by federal and state governments over the past 30 years to address this problem, rural provider distribution and shortage issues have persisted. In dermatology, though the workforce has risen in recent years (presently 3.4 per 100,000 population compared to 1.8 in 1965 and 2.8 in 1985), there remains a significant maldistribution toward economically thriving metropolitan areas and away from underserved areas (poor urban and rural) [21]. For specialty services like dermatology this means that many in remote areas who need treatment do not get it.

Teledermatology is one means by which these individuals can gain fair access to providers at a distance; however, the location and accessibility of telehealth may still be a problem because these units are typically nonmobile. This is a systemic problem and one of economics when considering who will take the responsibility of installing and maintaining the equipment when it is often hundreds of miles away from the systems and providers offering services.

For many elderly living in rural areas, getting to specialty healthcare is a significant problem. In 2000, 61 million Americans lived in rural areas and nearly 15% of the rural population was aged 65 years or older [22]. As they age the rural elderly confront multiple barriers to obtaining healthcare and there is a rising concern that those at greatest risk, including the elderly and those with chronic conditions, may not be able to obtain healthcare services due to geographic, physical, cognitive, or economic challenges. Telehealth technology may be a means to healthcare but logistics remains an issue and mobility is still often required to get to a telehealth site in some cases. Making telehealth services portable and available in the home has become a viable option for these individuals [23].

Persons aged 65 and over presently account for 12.5% of the population in the United States, but this figure is anticipated to grow significantly in the years to come [24]. By the year 2030, one in five Americans will be of age 65 or older. The very old (80 and over) is a demographic expected to have the greatest growth in the next quarter century and are at greatest risk for death and complications resulting from acute and chronic illness. It is estimated that 20% of the population, for the most part those with chronic illness, spend 80% of the healthcare dollar. It has also been found that healthcare during the last year of life constitutes 22% of all medical expenses (26% of Medicare, 18% of all non-Medicare, and 25% of Medicaid expenditures) for those aged 65 and over [25]. Healthcare has become increasingly expensive and complicated, at the same time efforts are being made to find cost-effective ways to care for patients with chronic medical conditions in less costly environments that are more appropriate and beneficial to the patient, especially in rural settings. But access remains an issue for those immobile or remotely located who cannot easily or effectively get to healthcare providers. Telehealth availability can, therefore, provide a means to primary and specialty care for those who do not have reasonable access.

The elderly have substantial medical dermatologic needs, a burden that increases in proportion to the size of the geriatric age group [26]. Potentially fatal skin diseases like malignant melanoma and cutaneous T-cell lymphoma appear with a dramatically increased incidence in older people, yet many in this frail demographic find it difficult to get appropriate dermatologic care and treatment due to functional debility and the inability to travel long distances. Skin conditions that rarely threaten life (nonhealing ulcers, dermatophytosis, seborrheic dermatitis, herpes zoster, xerosis, and pruritus) but compromise quality of life also occur frequently in older patients. In one study two-thirds of patients over the age of 65 and 83% of the octogenarians reported concern regarding their skin, with pruritus being the most frequent complaint [27]. Despite a high prevalence and long average duration of dermatologic concerns, very few of these patients consulted a physician. When examined, all subjects had at least one skin lesion, while symptomatic and/or medically significant disorders were present in about 65%. In addition a rapidly increasing number of older people seek dermatologic care for treatment and prevention of the effects of aging skin. Dermatologic conditions are frequent in the elderly, yet these patients often do not seek treatment, often due to functional impairment or geographic isolation.

With an aging population it would seem reasonable to place telehealth technology where the elderly are most likely to ultimately live – long-term care facilities. The ability to effectively address the dermatologic needs of residents in these facilities will become increasingly important as greater demands are placed on the healthcare system in the years to come, yet very few nursing homes have telehealth availability. In Missouri only one nursing home in the state has telehealth, allowing its residents to regularly utilize dermatology as well as other specialty services on site. This demand will increase. In 1995 about 0.6% of the U.S. population, or 1.5 million people, lived in 16,700 nursing homes, in which 1.8 million beds were maintained at 87% capacity [28]. By 2030 this number will have increased to 5 million [29, 30]. Ninety percent of nursing home residents are over the age of 65, most are female and white.

Most nursing home residents are debilitated, have a difficult time representing themselves autonomously, and need assistance with activities of daily living and instrumental activities of daily living, not to mention their dependency on care providers and family to ensure good follow-up and treatment of chronic health conditions. A sobering statistic is that nearly half of the people over the age of 65 will one day enter a nursing home, half of whom will stay at least a year and 21% at least 5 years [31]. Even more compelling is that 20% of U.S. deaths occur in nursing homes [32]. By 2030, when an estimated 20% of the population will be over the age of 65, there will have been a doubling of this demographic from 30 to 60 million people. The population over the age of 85 will also double from 3 to 6 million souls.

Evolving ethnic and cultural differences in patient populations is also becoming an increasingly important concern in terms of healthcare access. In 2003, 3.7 million people (11% of the older population) were foreign born, most from Europe and Latin America (35% each) and Asia (23%). In 2000, 13% of the older population spoke a language other than English at home, among them one-third spoke Spanish. Though the overall proportion of older people staying in nursing homes has fallen by 8% in recent years, the U.S. Census Bureau indicates that the proportion of black residents has increased while that of whites has decreased [33]. The Census Bureau projects that by 2030 the ethnic composition of the older population will have shifted to where 72% will be white, 11% Hispanic, 10% black, and 5% Asian. This is compared to 83%, 3%, 8%, and 6%, respectively, in 2003. How illness are interpreted and manifest in each of these groups, and the cultural mores that inform the response that patients and families will have to health concerns, will be increasingly important considerations for providers who are called upon to provide diagnosis and treatment services. Becoming sensitive to these needs and differences and becoming culturally competent is becoming an imperative for the good physician. Developing skills for tele-health specific to the needs of the elderly and ethnic groups who have been traditionally underserved will be doubly challenging considering the natural tendency to mistrust healthcare systems for many of these individuals.

Indeed, the need for innovative technologies that can bring specialized healthcare to a growing number of underserved will become a paramount concern in the years to come if systems and society are to remain committed to their obligation to care for vulnerable and disenfranchised persons whose health and welfare depend on their being able to seek healthcare where they are.

Burden and quality of life

One of the greatest barriers to the use of telehealth, or any new technology for that matter, is fear. For patients it is often the fear of intrusion or becoming distanced from their provider, and for providers it is being confronted with unfamiliar technology for which they may not have the knowledge or skills required for its use. Being sensitive and responsive to these concerns and to the human factors that impact utilization for both patients and other providers will be important for the present and future success of any telehealth or teledermatology program [34].

Almost every specialty has used telehealth in some way, though radiology, dermatology, and psychiatry/psychology have embraced it to a greater extent. For practitioners in specialties who have not been trained or traditionally worked in telehealth, there has historically been a reluctance to use it, often because of the discomfort of physically being separated from their patients. For dermatology this has been less of a problem because many training programs now incorporate one or both teledermatology functions, live-interactive or store-and-forward, into their training programs and practice. An increasing number of private dermatology practices also now utilize this technology.

For patients who are frail or with chronic conditions, the "perceived" burden of requiring them to interact via telehealth may be overwhelming and add to their burden of illness. These concerns may relate to their being overwhelmed by the technology itself or from the geographic and emotional distance they feel from their provider. Many patients however embrace telehealth once they become accustomed and encourage its use. Sometimes patients actually feel more satisfied and closer to their provider knowing they have more immediate access as a result of telehealth being available. In one cross-sectional survey study most dermatology outpatients were found to be accepting of the technologically and capable of participating in tele-dermatology interactions [35]. In other situations patients have been found to become frustrated when telehealth technology was not used more often because they had become convinced of its usefulness. This adds to the growing evidence that patients are becoming technologically sophisticated and interested in being more involved in their healthcare with a desire to have more control.

For patients living at home, and their caregivers, several potential obstacles to the receptiveness of using telehealth equipment have been identified, including maintaining home security, the potential for limiting the need for healthcare support, there being a very low or high degree of caregiver burden, and discomfort or disinterest in using the technology [36]. Often patients describe themselves as being "overwhelmed" when con-fronted by the use of telehealth technology, though in the long run they become quite satisfied with its use once they have had an opportunity to use it and become familiar with its benefits [37].

Exploitation

The development of telehealth over the past 20 years has offered a valuable contribution to healthcare providing new technical solutions and applica-tions that have a clear potential for becoming part of future practices. When new and exciting technology is introduced into a market system there is a natural tendency and a desire to market that technology. Healthcare pro-viders interested in the "new and fancy" glow of technology also may want to rapidly become skilled in its use and maximize its utility and may use it on as many patients as possible, regardless of whether skills are optimal or patients might benefit. Procedural interventions also tend to be reimbursed much more lucratively than evaluation and management services, thereby encouraging their use to maximize income, though to date reimbursement for teledermatology services, patient for patient, is the equivalent to in-person clinic visits.

Maximizing income from technology is not necessarily a bad thing, of course, as long as there is a clear clinical indication for its use, and patients are not being exploited in the interest of profit. It has been repeatedly shown that economic factors have statistically significant associations with the observed rate of utilization of healthcare technology in the United States [38]. From antibiotics to implantable defibrillators, MRI machines to endo-scopic exams … because we have it we tend to use it, and use it extensively, as long as it gets reimbursed. The traditional art combining diagnostic excellence with therapeutic and technological parsimony will be needed in the days to come as resources grow increasingly scarce and greater numbers require healthcare. The capacity to be parsimonious as a proceduralist specialty in the face of an emerging technology like telehealth will be a question that will challenge the experts for many years to come.

When the use of technology becomes a self-fulfilling prophecy, whereby it is now *profit* centered rather than *patient* centered, and income and profit become the driving force of clinical decision making, then the ethical bounds of our profession have been exceeded. At that moment the technological imperative transforms the healing profession into a healthcare enterprise and our patients become a means to an end. However, the ongoing development of standards, both technical and clinical, for teledermatology will help to mitigate this risk and should lead to limiting teledermatology care delivery to that which is of high clinical and technical quality, provided by highly trained and competent providers.

Conclusion

The expansive development and ongoing deployment of telehealth and other forms of information and communication technologies is rapidly changing the landscape of healthcare, both for the inpatient setting and in the community. As specialized providers skilled in the use of telehealth, dermatologists must remain committed to and driven by the same moral precepts and ethical traditions that define their role as healthcare professionals. They must be committed to compassionately defining and seeking the best possible outcome for their patients, remain honest and fair in the treatment of patients, and utilize resources honestly and prudently. Kenneth Iserson [39] has proposed an ethical code for telehealth practitioners to serve as a normative guide in the use of this still-evolving technology: the code pledges commitment to benevolent action, fairness, integrity, respect for others, avoiding harm, pursuing sound scholarship, and insuring appropriate oversight. These are virtuous attributes of any healthcare provider but are of particular importance to those using new and evolving technologies that have economic impact and the potential to both help and harm. Telehealth, and in particular teledermatology, are interventions that have a huge potential for doing good primarily because they have the capacity to diagnose and treat many who may otherwise go unserved. How we as individuals, systems, and society deploy and promote access to these services will be reflective of our moral framework, as well as the professional intent and means by which we selflessly serve the most vulnerable.

It should also be remembered that telehealth is an enabling tool to enhance the delivery of overall healthcare. When used correctly in the appropriate setting, it can have a tremendous positive impact for our patients. Its goal, however, is not to replace the shared trust, comfort, and compassion that are manifest by the healing touch of a physician.

REFERENCES

[1] Stanberry B. Telemedicine: Barriers and opportunities in the 21st century, *J Int Med* 2000;247:615–28.

[2] Fleming D. The ethical challenges of new technology. *Eur J Med Res* 2002;7 (Suppl 1):25.

[3] Comford T, Klecun-Debrowska E. Ethical perspectives in evaluation of telehealth. *Camb Q Healthc Ethics* 2001;10(2):161–9.

[4] Bauer K. Home based telemedicine: A survey of ethical issues. *Camb Q Healthc Ethics* 2001;10(2):137–46.

[5] Bauer K. The ethical and social dimensions of home-based telemedicine. *Crit Rev Biomed Eng* 2000;28(3 and 4):541–4.

[6] Ashley R. Telemedicine: Legal, ethical and liability considerations. *J Am Dietetic Assoc* 2002;102(2):267–9.

[7] Grigsby J, Sanders J. Telemedicine: Where it is and where it's going. *Ann Int Med* 1998;129(2):123–7.

[8] Butler D. Informed consent and patient videotaping. *Acad Med* 2002;77 (2):184–91.

[9] Stanberry B. The legal and ethical aspects of telemedicine. 3: Telemedicine and malpractice. *J Telemed Telecare* 1998;4(2):72–9.

[10] Irvine R. Mediating telemedicine: Ethics at a distance. *Int Med J* 2005;35:56–8.

[11] Silverman J. Would a virtual office visit cut long waits, paperwork? An end to true "medicine"? *Fam Pract News* 2003;33:53.

[12] Evans H. "High tech vs high touch": The impact of medical technology on patient care. In J Clare, R Allman (eds), *Sociomedical perspectives on patient care*. Lexington, Kentucky: University Press of Kentucky, 1993, pp. 83–95.

[13] Finnish Medical Association. *Ethical guidelines in telemedicine*. 1997. www:// laakarilitto.fi/e/ethics/telemed/html Last accessed on July 11, 2003.

[14] Bredfeldt R, Ripani A, Cuddeback G. The effect of touch on patients' estimates of time in the waiting and examination rooms. *Fam Med* 1987;19(4):299–302.

[15] Fleming D, Boren S, Alber S, et al. Internal medicine telehealth training and evaluation project (IMTTEP). *Telemed eHealth* 2006;12(2):210.

[16] Miller E. Telemedicine and doctor-patient communication: An analytical survey of the literature. *J Telemed Telecare* 2001;7:1–17.

[17] Demiris G, Oliver D, Fleming D, Edison K. Hospice staff attitudes towards telehospice. *Am J Hospice Palliat Care*. 2004;21(5):343–7.

[18] U.S. Bureau of Census. Income, poverty, and health insurance coverage in the United States: 2005. Current Population Reports Series P 60-231. Washington, DC: U.S. Printing Office, 2006.

[19] Marmot M. Inequalities in health care. *NEJM* 2001;345(2):134–6.

[20] Hart LG, Salsberg E, Phillips DM, Lishner DM. Rural health care providers in the United States. *J Rural Health* 2002;18 Suppl:211–32.

[21] Resneck J. Too few or too many dermatologists? *Arch Dermatol* 2001;137: 1293–301.

[22] Rosenthal T, Fox C. Access to health care for the rural elderly. *JAMA* 2000;284: 2034–6.

[23] Fleming D, Demiris G, Edison K. The value of Telehomecare for the frail elderly. *Telemed E Health* 2003;9 (Suppl 1):S-102.

[24] U.S. Bureau of the Census. Decennial census of population, 1900–1980 and projections of populations of the United States: 1982–2050. Current Population Reports Series P-25, no. 922. Washington, DC: U.S. Bureau of the Census, 2006.

[25] Hoover D, Crystal S, Kumar, Sambamoorthi U, and Cantor J. Medical expenditures during the last year of life: Findings from the 1992–1996 Medicare Current Beneficiary Survey. *Health Serv Res* 2002;37(6):1625–42.

[26] Kosmadaki M, Gilchrest B. The demographics of aging the United States. *Arch Dermatol* 2002;138:1427–8.

[27] Beauregard S, Gilchrest B. A survey of skin problems and care regimens in the elderly. *Arch Dermatol* 1987;123(12):1638–43.

[28] Gabrel C, Jones A. The National Nursing Home Survey: 1995 summary. *Vital Health Stat 13*. 2000;146:1–83.

[29] Zedlewski SR, Barnes RO, Burt MK, McBride TD, Meyer J. *The needs of the elderly in the 21st century*. Washington, DC: The Urban Institute, 1989.

[30] Doty PJ. The oldest old and the use of institutional long-term care from an international perspective. In R Suzman, DP Willis, KG Manton (eds), *The oldest old*. New York: Oxford University Press, 1992, pp. 251–67.

[31] Kemper P, Murtaugh CM. Lifetime use of nursing home care. *NEJM* 1991;324:595–600.

[32] Ersek M, Wilson S. The challenges and opportunities in providing end-of-life care in nursing homes. *J Palliat Med* 2003;6(1):45–57.

[33] 65+ in the United States: 2005. U.S. Census Bureau Report. Issued December 2005.

[34] Demiris G, Edison K, Sridhar S, Patrick T, Fleming D. Human factors in implementing telemedicine programs: Part 2. *Telemed eHealth* 2004;10 (Suppl 1):S-58.

[35] Qureshi A, Kvedar J. Patient knowledge and attitude toward information technology and teledermatology: Some tentative findings. *Telemed J E Health* 2003;9(3):259–64.

[36] Buckley K, Tran B, Prandoni C. Receptiveness, use and acceptance of telehealth by caregivers of stroke patients in the home. Online *J Issues Nurs* 2004; 9(3). http://nursingworld.org/ojin/topic16/tpc16_6.htm

[37] Whitten P, Doolittle G, Mackert M. Telehospice in Michigan: Use and patient acceptance. *Am J Hospice Palliat Med* 2004;21(3):191–5.

[38] Rasool A, Xue L. Variations in the utilization of medical technology as influenced by socio-economic factors in the case of magnetic resonance imaging (MRI). *Int J Healthc Tech Mgmt* 2000;2(1–4):337–57.

[39] Iserson K. Telemedicine: A proposal for an ethical code. *Camb Q Healthc Ethics* 2000:9:404–6.

10 Teledermatology in dermatology residency

Anne E. Burdick, Kimberly A. Sackheim, and Daniel Siegel

In recent years, several dermatology residency programs in the United States have incorporated teledermatology as part of their training programs. Some programs use store-and-forward (S/F) systems, such as the Brooke Army Medical Center (BAMC), the State University of New York (SUNY) Downstate, and the Jackson Memorial Hospital (JMH) program at the Miller University of Miami (UM) School of Medicine. Other residency programs utilize live-interactive videoconferencing (LIV) systems including the University of Missouri – Columbia (UMC) School of Medicine. In S/F consults, senior residents typically conduct the initial patient assessment by evaluating the patient history and images from a secure web site followed by a faculty member who reviews the case, edits the draft consultation, and submits the final version to the web site. In LIV dermatology visits, a resident interviews and examines the patient with a videoconferencing system and then presents the case to the faculty attending as would occur in a traditional clinic setting. The faculty dermatologist then interviews and examines the patient with the videoconferencing equipment and provides recommendations to the remote site with a medical chart maintained at the academic center.

A good example of how LIV teledermatology is integrated into a residency program is seen at the University of Missouri's Department of Dermatology. The teledermatology clinic is not a separate method of care delivery; rather it is integrated into the everyday way dermatology is practiced and is part of the regular day-to-day clinic operation in the residency program. Two exam rooms in the university dermatology clinic are equipped with state-of-the-art videoconferencing systems. In this program, underserved rural patients have been cared for via teledermatology with resident participation since 2001. While live videoconferencing alone was used in the early years, now a hybrid model is used that capitalizes on the best of both S/F and LIV teledermatology. Patients are seen in two hybrid teledermatology half day clinics per week; one is a general and the other a pediatric teledermatology clinic. High-quality digital photos are seen either before or concomitantly with the patient visit. This adds standardization and decreases the need for perfect video camera control at every patient site, while allowing live interaction with the patient so that further history and physical exam as needed, as well as patient and sometime referring provider education, may be accomplished. Residents see patients just as they do in-person, with residents gradually taking on more patient care and education responsibility as they progress through the residency program. As new teledermatology sites are opened throughout rural Missouri, the residents routinely see dermatology diseases in advanced stages of neglect.

Since 1998, the UM has provided S/F teledermatology consultations to Project Outreach, an HIV/AIDS Clinic in Florida City, Florida. The Project Outreach referring physician notifies his nurse manager that a patient requires a dermatology consult. The nurse then captures digital images of the involved skin and enters the patient's history onto the secure server. The UM Telemedicine Program administrator is notified by email of pending S/F consults and he then emails and pages the second- or third-year resident on the teledermatology rotation. This resident evaluates the clinical information and digital images on the server. The resident then drafts a diagnosis or differential diagnosis, with the workup and therapeutic recommendations stored on the server. A designated faculty member then reviews the case and the resident's draft consult making any edits before signing off on the final version. The residents are then able to review the final consult for their education. This has been tremendously valuable to the residents as they see not only the comments and changes from the staff but also how they articulate and manage the patients. In some cases, the entire recommendation is deleted and a new set of recommendations result. The resident is able to compare what he or she had written and what the staff has documented. Of note, supervising staff style and variability becomes more evident to the resident physicians in the teledermatology process.

The diagnoses that residents have seen from Project Outreach ranged widely from solitary lesions such as dermal nevi, seborrheic keratoses, and Kaposi's sarcoma to eruptions such as contact dermatitis, atopic dermatitis, herpes zoster, and secondary syphilis. Biopsies are performed at Project Outreach by a nurse practitioner, who was trained in shave and punch biopsies at JMH prior to the start of the teledermatology program. Pathology reports are sent to the referring physician and if there are questions, a follow-up query is posed either by a telephone call or a second teleconsultation.

A former JMH Dermatology chief resident at the UM, Tami deAraujo, MD, stated,

Teledermatology is definitely a unique way of practicing our profession. Because the physicians are limited in their ability to exam the patient, the exercise of differential diagnosis and management algorithms becomes paramount. To me, that is the greatest learning tool that teledermatology provides. Besides the academic benefits, I think another positive is the satisfaction one gets in being able to help a patient that otherwise would have no access to care. In short, I think it's a valid experience for the physician and a great service to the community it serves.

Teledermatology training received by two graduates of the JMH Dermatology residency program was a useful experience since they are now providing teledermatology consults as part of their private practice responsibilities in multispecialty groups. One graduate practices in Montana where one afternoon a week he uses a LIV system to evaluate patients. Another graduate works in a remote area of Maine and was asked during his job interview about his familiarity with telemedicine since it would be part of his clinical responsibilities.

Two other medical centers that have integrated S/F teledermatology into their dermatology training programs are the BAMC and the SUNY Downstate. Both have had similar experiences, perhaps somewhat unexpected, related to the educational impact teledermatology has had on their training programs. BAMC in San Antonio, Texas, was one of the first teledermatology programs to incorporate teledermatology into its residency program. As with any academic program, residents had been assessed on a regular basis using formal tools (tests, in service examinations) and informal tools (daily staff supervision and presentation). Using these traditional methods, each staff formulates his or her opinion about the quality of a given resident and their strengths and weaknesses based on interactions occurring during a few months of each year. This assessment is typically used to observe and strengthen those areas using various subtle and not so subtle tools (e.g., the tradition of questioning residents about their knowledge base during rounds). Once the S/F teledermatology program BAMC was integrated, we found that residents who were very knowledgeable, nonetheless, had knowledge gaps that were not exposed using the traditional assessment methods. During resident supervision, numerous staff noted that residents were not picking up certain common findings in the images or had ignored an important part of the history when recommending a medication (e.g., history indicated that patient did not respond to that medication at presentation). When this trend was noted by most of the staff dermatologists supervising senior residents, we explored why this might be the case.

It became clear that what we do during staff supervision during clinic is not a completely independent and objective assessment of residents' knowledge. Several things occur that do not allow for an objective measurement of the resident presenting the case. First, the history from the patient changes slightly with time. In addition, the residents are very quick to pick up on our cues when presenting the patient to staff dermatologist. Most staff make gestures inadvertently or advertently (rolling of eyes, pursing the lips, frowning, smiling, nodding, etc.) when listening to the presentation by the resident. The resident then is able to assess the gestures and will either broaden the differential or management plan or go to an entirely different plan. This, of course, is not inherently negative behavior; however, this makes an unbiased assessment very difficult. In the end, it is difficult to determine if the resident would have come up with the same diagnosis or management plan independent of the staff's involvement. S/F teledermatology essentially changes the paradigm of staff supervision. The resident is forced to take the information provided by teledermatology and come up with a best diagnosis and management plan. Unlike a routine outpatient record, the resident has to write a recommendation as he or she would in an inpatient consultation and explicitly articulate the thought process and the management plan that explicitly discusses an algorithmic approach to the treatment (e.g., if the patient does not improve with the first set of recommendations, the second set of recommendations will include . . . , etc.).

With teledermatology, the staff dermatologist is reviewing a completed diagnosis and management plan that has been unaltered by staff input to that point. The resident is forced to articulate a completed thought process of how a diagnosis was derived and how this patient should be managed, not only initially, but also over a longer time frame. This is because the tele-dermatologist is providing contingency plans for the referring clinician, in case the patient does not improve.

While the impetus for the teledermatology program at BAMC was to assist with workload issues, the staff at BAMC realized that our traditional education/supervision methodology needed to be improved to ensure that the gaps of knowledge were identified earlier in the residency for remediation or correction. This was a somewhat unexpected outcome of the program, but one that may have a great impact on dermatology training programs.

The educational experiences found at the SUNY Downstate are very similar to those at BAMC. At SUNY Downstate, two different approaches to telemedicine are being used. Working with Project Renewal (http://www.projectrenewal.org/) and using TeleDerm Solutions, Inc.[R] ASP software, dermatology care is offered to inner city homeless people getting primary care in a mobile clinic or individuals living in Project Renewal's shelter. The Project Renewal primary care provider enters the data and the tele-dermatology resident and attending are notified via email that a consult is pending. The resident answers the consult and the attending then reviews and annotates it and sends it back. This has been an intellectually rewarding process for the dermatologists, primary care providers, and patients. Patients in need of a hands-on evaluation and treatment by a dermatologist are either seen in a Project Renewal site or at Kings County Hospital.

The second approach at SUNY Downstate involves the use of cellphone cameras, where the resident on the consultation service and the attending physician each have a Sprint PM-8920 (the first cameraphone with true megapixel imaging capability) with an LED "flash" and a primitive optical macro mode. Patients are seen by residents and photographs are taken after consent is obtained. For urgent consultations (when attendings are not immediately available for in-person supervision), photographs are transmitted to the on-call dermatologist and cases are discussed by telephone with a staff physician regarding appropriate management. All patients are seen in person by an attending physician within 24 hr (per hospital regulations). To test the accuracy of this teleconsultation system, over a dozen consecutive cases were presented as "unknowns" to 9 attending staff and 14 residents both with and without accompanying history. Concordance between histology, onsite evaluation, and camera images was very high. The data is being analyzed with plans for publishing a larger series.

A similar model of S/F teledermatology exists at the University of Missouri's residency program. Urgent patients in the hospital, in the emergency department, and in the urgent care clinic are evaluated by dermatology residents who, with permission, obtain high-quality digital images which are sent to the on-call attending dermatologist through an internal secure email link. The patient is then discussed over the telephone and treatment decisions and follow-up plans are made. Patients are then seen in person by the attending dermatologist (if hospitalized) or in follow up in the dermatology clinic. Currently, reimbursement is not sought for patients not seen in-person.

Like the experience at the BAMC, occasionally attending dermatologists found that the residents at SUNY have gaps in dermatologic knowledge that were not detected in the past using traditional evaluations, but were identified when reviewing teledermatology consults. Again, the spoken and unspoken cues received by the resident from the staff dermatologist during a presentation are thought to result in a revision of their presentations. On the other hand, the S/F draft consultation provides a definitive independent product based on the resident's experience and knowledge.

Residents are uniformly intrigued by challenges to make a diagnosis and recommendation based on a limited standardized history and a limited image set. The challenges for residents are the same as those for the faculty dermatologists in using S/F teledermatology:

1. inability to palpate the skin or skin lesion;
2. inability to ask additional questions (however, many do call patients on the phone to get additional information, if necessary);
3. inability to perform office-based tests (potassium hydroxide wet mounts for diagnosing yeast infections, Tzanck preparations to assess for viral infections, etc.);
4. limited view of the skin and skin condition(s) imposed by imaging.

In using teledermatology, the residents begin to develop experience and confidence in making clinical diagnoses without potassium hydroxide wet mounts to confirm Candida or fungal infectious or Tzanck preparations to confirm varicella-herpes infections. In essence, the staff dermatologists have found that the cognitive abilities of the residents actually increase when you limit the information and tests. The residents also learn to write treatment plans that are written in an algorithm form where initial therapy is offered and a second or third alternative plan is also given if the original therapy is unsuccessful. This is different from a routine dermatology patient recommendation in which the patient is asked to make a follow-up appointment to determine how the patient is responding to therapy. This is a very significant component of the evaluation as it provides the thought process of the resident to the supervising staff in ways that were not done in traditional supervision model.

Teledermatology adds a new facet to resident education and provides a unique tool to objectively assess dermatology house staff. Training in tele-medicine improves our compliance with three of the required core com-petencies of the Accreditation Council for Graduate Medical Education (ACGME). These three competencies are

1. the "practice-based learning" competency that encompasses knowl-edge about the use of information technology and improvements of patient care;
2. the "system-based practice" competency that pertains to an under-standing of cost-effectiveness and patient advocacy;
3. the "professionalism" competency that is addressed in the manner in which the resident communicates with the referring physician.

For many years, the American Board of Dermatology has used images to assess the diagnostic and cognitive abilities of graduating residents. The inservice and certifying examinations now have become online tests and contain a significant amount of images as part of the evaluation. Therefore, it is not surprising that teledermatology has had tremendous success as an educational tool for residents. The authors speculate that S/F tele-dermatology may be an "oral exam" equivalent to other specialties in which your thought process and your cognitive ability to approach a problem are assessed rather than determining your knowledge of a given disease or ability to detect a given finding. Although, more studies are needed, it is becoming clear that teledermatology could be used as an additional tool in certifying oral board examinations and could provide an additional objec-tive measurement of residents' knowledge.

In conclusion, teledermatology is becoming an important educational experience for dermatology residents and can provide a useful assessment tool for resident competency in dermatology. The most common way resi-dents are evaluated by faculty dermatologists is by the faculty recalling perceived strengths, major recurring issues, and gaps in knowledge. With S/F teledermatology, residents must change the way they approach a skin condition:

1. They are forced to document their thought processes for determining the diagnosis and management plan.
2. They need to document their diagnosis and a stepwise treatment plan tailored to the primary care provider.
3. Residents are required to design a contingency treatment plan for patients in an algorithm format for a one-time consultation (e.g., "If no

change after 2 weeks, change to ...") compared to an immediate plan (e.g., "follow up in 4 weeks").
4. Residents must learn to utilize available references other than immediate staff feedback and thereby increase their knowledge base.

S/F consultations offer limited visual images with which to formulate a diagnosis and management plan compared with a live patient interaction. Additionally, S/F consultations are completed by resident physicians without immediate staff feedback. This format allows for an independent assessment of resident competency. S/F consultations provide a different insight into a resident's diagnostic thought process, therapeutic decisions, and management plans than does a clinic-based encounter.

In addition, LIV and S/F teledermatology allow resident dermatology physicians access to patients who would not otherwise receive expert dermatological care, rural and urban underserved patients in the United States, as well as potentially millions of underserved dermatology patients worldwide. A wide variety of cutaneous pathology and exposure to all racial and ethnic groups may be accessed from training programs anywhere in the world. The legal, regulatory, and logistical barriers to such access are currently being addressed.

Finally, teledermatology has the added benefit of adding to collections of teaching cases that can be used during a residency program. Overall, teledermatology provides an additional means for resident physicians to develop their diagnostic and management skills and a means of staff dermatologists to make better assessments of their knowledge base. It seems likely that a very positive outcome, and one that was somewhat unexpected, is an improvement in the training of our resident dermatologists with teledermatology.

11 Art of teledermatology

Karen E. Edison and Hon S. Pak

Introduction

As with every professional aspect of medicine there is both science and art involved in the practice of teledermatology. While the evidence shows that, compared to in-person care, we generally make the same diagnosis and recommend the same treatment using teledermatology, technology's impact on the "art" of practicing dermatology has been less well described. The art of teledermatology, in many respects, is equally important as the scientific considerations. Referring clinicians, patients, and teledermatologists that are uncomfortable or dissatisfied with the teledermatology consult process can prevent a teledermatology program from being successful regardless of the scientific evidence that supports its use.

This chapter will address the art of teledermatology as it applies to both live-interactive and store-and-forward teledermatology. These two modalities are discussed separately since various factors (e.g., differences in dermatologist-patient interactivity) influence how the teledermatology consult is managed by the teledermatologist.

Store-and-forward teledermatology

The finite dataset and store-and-forward teledermatology

There are notable differences in how we manage skin conditions and practice clinic-based dermatology compared to how we practice store-and-forward teledermatology. A major departure from live-interactive teledermatology revolves around the fact that the dermatologist and the patient (with rare exceptions) do not interact with one another. We should also acknowledge that most of what we do in traditional dermatology consists of managing referrals and not consultations. Store-and-forward teledermatology, for the most part, is truly a consultation service. A consultative service implies that the teledermatologist is only making recommendations and that the referring provider remains responsible for managing the patient. This may include writing prescriptions, ordering tests, providing education, performing a procedure, and the like. Practicing store-and-forward teledermatologists believe that the cognitive component of dermatology is emphasized when using teledermatology. This is because the consultant has a finite set of data and no ability to interact directly with the patient, a situation that forces the consultant to use all of his or her cognitive skills to arrive at a diagnosis and provide a management plan.

What to expect

Teledermatologists should not settle for suboptimal information or images. Nonetheless, this author is amazed at the ability of physicians to take limited set of information and dynamically use our other senses to obtain a more complete picture. If, for example, the history of the patient is not consistent, we tend to leverage our visual findings to derive a diagnosis or management plan. What should you expect as a teledermatologist? The following list describes the important features of a teledermatology consultation:

1. Standardized set of history (chief complaint, onset, symptoms, course history, location, previous treatment, allergies, current medications).
2. Standardized set of images (image protocol based on anatomic location(s))
   a) Example
      i) Rash on right elbow requires evaluation of a standard view of knees, elbows, and examination of scalp
      ii) Rash on hands requires examination of feet
   b) Close ups (12 in.)
      i) Perpendicular and standardized to ensure resolution is adequate.
3. Quality of images
   a) Focus
   b) Lesions clearly identifiable
   c) Lighting.

What is expected of the teledermatologist

The expectations of the teledermatologist depend on the role you are playing (referral vs consultation); however, there are some basic principles to follow. First, you must have insight into the people who are sending you the consults, their capabilities, and their limitations. For example, most referring providers do not have the capability to perform or interpret a skin scraping. In addition, they may not have the instruments or supplies necessary to do some common procedures such as shave or punch biopsies or cryotherapy. Moreover, there may be issues on the local formulary that may restrict what you can recommend or prescribe for treatment. Last, it is important that you understand the motivation or incentives to perform these tests or procedures.

When you are answering the consults or making recommendations, we recommend that you consider the following:

1. *Diagnosis*: Do not list a long differential diagnosis for a condition when you really already know the diagnosis. For example, if the patient has vitiligo then call it vitiligo and do not list leprosy, syphilis, and other unrelated diagnosis unless it is appropriate. It may appear as though we are not sure of the diagnosis. A useful rule is, if you would not list differential diagnoses for an in-person visit, then do not list it for tele-dermatology. When listing differential diagnoses, you should prioritize your list, explain the order, and provide a logical approach as much as possible.

2. *Work ups*: Understand if and how these tests are handled at each referring sites (KOH [potassium hydroxide] preparation, Tzanck preparation, Gram stain, etc.). Note that in-office tests, especially KOH, are rarely done. When they are performed, the interpretation should be questioned unless you have information to the contrary. In general, we should assume that KOH and other in office tests are not available and make recommendations based on not being able to do these tests. For example, for a hand rash (with a differential diagnosis of tinea manuum), consider treating the rash with antifungal cream for 2 weeks then fluocinonide ointment 0.05% TID for 2 weeks.

3. *Treatments*: Use generic medications whenever possible since availability of dermatologic medications may be limited and variable. You should not assume that referring providers know about the recommended medications and their common side effects. You should be explicit on medication name and its use/directions. If there are any special instructions, please include them for the provider/patient (examples include tretinoin or fluorouracil use). When evidence shows no significant difference between a procedural vs pharmacologic management, consider using medications over a procedure (cryotherapy vs fluorouracil or imiquimod). In addition, we generally recommend a step-by-step management plan. (For example, try A for X duration then go to B for X duration then reconsult via tele-dermatology or refer to dermatologist if no improvement.) In some cases, empiric treatments may be appropriate without having the luxury to confirm the diagnosis with a test.

4. *Procedures*: Most providers are not well trained on common dermatologic procedures or may not have the facility to perform them efficiently. Be able to refer the patient to local dermatologist or surgeon if available. (Other specialties that routinely perform procedures include general surgeons or podiatrists.) You could also consider training local

referring providers or physician extenders during visits or at your location when feasible or appropriate.

5. *Follow ups*: We as dermatologists arguably tend to have patients follow up with us more frequently then needed in many cases. Most follow ups can and should be done by the referring provider. Advise them about what to look for and what to do if the patient does not respond appropriately. We should develop relationships with dermatologists near the referring locations in cases where a referral becomes necessary (Moh's surgery or laser). As indicated above, follow up can be with other procedure-based specialty (general surgery, podiatry, plastic surgery, etc.) as appropriate. Many follow ups can be scheduled as needed (PRN). If the patient does not improve, teledermatology can, and should, be used for follow up if you need to see the case again.

6. *Patient/provider education*: Teledermatology provides a wonderful opportunity to educate both the patient and the referring provider, but there must be a balance of quality of content vs length. We should be mindful of how much time providers have to read your recommendations or education, and simply copying and pasting canned, lengthy notes on conditions tend to be ineffectual. When possible and appropriate, try to customize the education to the provider and the patient for the given condition. Use Internet links to information when possible for more in-depth discussions to give provider and patient the option to do further research.

7. *What if additional information is needed whether it is suboptimal images or history?* We should never compromise patient safety and should ask for additional images (e.g., image of worrisome pigmented lesions) when we cannot reasonably be confident of our diagnosis or management. This will vary based on the experience of the consultant. You must provide feedback informally to improve the quality of images and history to ensure that the referring sites understand your standards. On the other hand, do not ask for additional images unless you truly cannot make a diagnosis. For example, if only one of the two images is blurry, and the other image is good enough for you to make the diagnosis, then we should not ask for additional photos. You can always call the patient or referring provider if it will expedite this consult. Spending a few minutes with a patient on the phone clarifying a history may make a significant difference on your diagnosis or management.

Issues to avoid in store-and-forward teledermatology

1. *Avoid being judgmental*: It is inappropriate to use adjectives that either place or highlight blame on the referring provider. Stick with neutral/factual information and try to make helpful recommendations. Avoid statements that can be perceived as being overly critical or judgmental.

2. *Teledermatology is a formal report*: Many teledermatologists tend to be initially too informal or conversational in the recommendation section. Note that this is a formal report and part of the medical record.

3. *Avoid writing for medications that are unavailable*: Use generic formulations to the extent possible. Keep in mind that many places have limited formularies. Therefore, try to avoid uncommon products when more readily available products are an adequate substitute. Also, designate whether a medication is OTC or if it is a new brand medication. When prescribing a medication, provide specifics so the primary care provider (PCP) can write the prescription correctly, especially regarding duration of treatment. Some primary care physicians are registered to prescribe isotretinoin (Accutane) through the iPledge program, but most are not.

4. *Others*: Articulate your thought process in how and why you derived at your diagnosis and differential diagnosis. Do not assume that the referring provider knows the diagnosis but do not deliver diagnostic information in a condescending manner (e.g., "any physician would know that this represents..."). Show confidence but not arrogance. Develop a relationship with your referring providers. Call and visit the referring provider when possible, and contact the provider if there is something urgent or sensitive that would be better handled via person to person or if additional information is needed. Last, always thank the referring provider for their service.

The art of live-interactive teledermatology

Establishment of the healing relationship

Because in live-interactive teledermatology the dermatologist and patient interact directly, the initial and perhaps most crucial step to solidifying the clinical moment is to engender trust and inspire confidence by putting the patient at ease. This can be aided by scanning the entire room where the teledermatologist is located to show the patient exactly who is in the room. Small talk and the use of humor can also help ease the tension and help the teledermatologist to virtually "reach" across the video screen, "touch" the patient, and establish the human connection needed for a therapeutic doctor/patient relationship. Most children and adults enjoy being on the video screen once they understand the process. Patients also appreciate that healthcare is being brought to them and are grateful that they can receive the care they need without long, expensive, inconvenient, and often debilitating drives. Patients may likewise take the initiative of accessing their providers via telehealth having learned the value and convenience of this venue and once they have established a trusting relationship.

Example case – This live-interactive teledermatologist cared for an 86-year-old female with bullous pemphigoid at a distance of 100 miles for several years. When the patient was dying from other causes, she made a teledermatology appointment specifically to say goodbye to the teledermatologist with whom she had a warm therapeutic healing relationship even though they were never physically together.

Technical issues

Careful attention to good eye contact is essential. If the teledermatologist is sitting too close to the video screen and the camera is located above the screen, it may appear to the patient that the dermatologist is looking down towards the floor, which can be disconcerting for the patient and make the physician look inattentive and unconcerned about the patient. Every opportunity to express openness, comfort, and trust are to be optimized at a distance. A space of approximately 8 ft is needed between the examining physician and the camera in order to achieve the appearance of good eye contact, thus counterbalancing the necessary elevation of the camera.

Careful attention to the microphone is also important. Today's microphones are extremely sensitive and can pick up the faintest of sounds, including whispers. While it is possible to mute the microphone on the provider end, a policy of not discussing issues in the videoconferencing room that one would not want the patient to hear is advised. The loudness and pitch of the speaker's voice should also be considered. Sensitive microphones make it unnecessary to raise one's voice when using live-interactive technology. While new users may be inclined to raise their voices when they first start using a live-interactive system, speaking in a normal voice is all that is required.

If the video examination is not adequate for confident dermatological diagnosis, the operator of the camera on site may need gentle coaching. Helping the camera operator to switch between the "overhead" video camera and the "close-up" camera may be necessary. Rarely, the consulting physician may need to take over operation of the camera on site, which is now possible with modern systems. If lack of focus is a problem, it will help to place an object with a sharp edge (such as a piece of paper) in the field of an autofocus camera to help it focus. If the image quality is still not adequate, the teledermatologist should request that the personnel on site with the patient take and project a series of high-quality digital photos of the patient's skin condition. Having a hybrid system with this capacity is useful. While high-quality digital photos aid in diagnosis, having videoconferencing available at the same time allows the teledermatologist to ask the patient follow-up questions and obtain additional information, either from the patient or from the physical examination, if needed.

Other technical problems may include dropped calls and problems with the video and/or audio system. Having the phone number of the technical team on hand at all times is advised. In the course of a live-interactive teledermatology clinic setting, one may need to leave one patient site while technical problems are being resolved, see a patient in another site, and then return to the original site to see the original patient. Partnering and securing a close working relationship with the skilled personnel caring for the patient on site is important to keep the patient from becoming frustrated and to keep the healing relationship sound so effective communication and trust are not lost when disruptions occur due to technological delays.

Management of clinical uncertainty

After making optimum use of the available technology there may on rare occasions still be a need to see the patient in person. Careful questioning will reveal the patient's readiness and capability of traveling for dermatological care. Some patients will be able and willing, while others will find it very difficult. Understanding the resources available in the patient's vicinity is very important. If the patient cannot travel for a face-to-face visit and if there is a provider locally who is proficient in biopsy techniques, referral for biopsy may be in the patient's best interest in the face of clinical uncertainty.

If biopsies are done by another provider off site, a clear understanding as to whom the biopsy specimen is sent is crucial. Depending on the clinical situation, such as with inflammatory dermatoses, it will be helpful for the teledermatologist to provide the pre-op differential diagnosis including the spelling of all words. In return, it is always useful to also have a detailed microscopic description, if not a recut of the biopsy, sent to the teledermatologist.

Example case – This teledermatologist recently saw a frail 81-year-old white male 150 miles away with a lentigo simplex of his right nasal bridge. It was slightly darker and slightly more irregular than the teledermatologist was willing to accept and call it a benign lesion. On gentle questioning, it was clear that this patient and his wife could not travel for care. Consequently, a high-quality digital photo was requested and sent to the dermatologist and the patient will be followed via teledermatology in 3 months to ensure that this lesion is not changing. The patient expressed relief and was comfortable with the plan of careful observation by the teledermatologist.

Other office-based laboratory tests, such KOH examinations and mineral oil preparations, may be unavailable in some off-site settings. The teledermatologist may sometimes feel compelled to treat based on clinical judgment without the usual laboratory confirmations to which they are accustomed. A learning curve for new users can also be expected as confidence with the technology grows.

Most experienced live-interactive teledermatologists report that compared to in-person care, they use slightly different data inputs in clinical decision making. The patient's history may become a little more important and most will compensate for the lack of true "touch" capacity by asking on-site personnel to feel or pinch the skin. Induration and firmness can be evaluated by watching this occur and by asking the on-site provider and the patient to describe. Cutaneous scalp disorders can be particularly challenging and may require shaving off the hair surrounding the lesion in order to get an excellent image. Scaling skin diseases can sometimes be better evaluated by wetting the skin for a second view. Color may be altered if the light and background are not standardized in all patient settings. If there is any question, a variety of views with different light settings can be helpful. Simply having a digital photo taken will give a slightly different view and important additional clinical information.

Relations with on-site providers

In some clinical settings, the patient's PCP may be present during the examination of their patient. Excellent consultant etiquette is needed in this situation. Careful explanation to the patient about his or her skin pathology and its treatment can also be helpful for the PCP to hear. If at all possible, genuinely complimenting the PCP on the patient's management up to the time of the teledermatology visit will engender collegial feelings as well. If a procedure needs to be performed, offering to supervise via video may be very useful in garnering the confidence of both the patient and their PCP. If the PCP agrees to perform the procedure and indicates comfort with doing it, it will still be important to offer specific instructions about the equipment needed and the mechanics of the procedure.

Example case – This teledermatologist recently diagnosed granuloma annulare in a 42-year-old white female 400 miles away in an underserved area. The patient's PCP was a clinical nurse practitioner and she was present with the patient during the teledermatology visit. The patient was distressed by the appearance of the granuloma annulare on her hands and forearms. A decision was made to treat with intralesional steroid medication. A careful explanation about the size of the needle, the concentration of the steroid mixture, and the placement of the needle in the skin were offered to the CNP. An offer to watch and assist virtually was declined and the patient was treated successfully by the CNP.

Follow up with the referring provider

Follow up with the referring provider for telehealth services does not differ for that required for in-person care. Having an electronic medical record (EMR) shared between the two clinical sites allows the dermatologist to enter a note into the EMR that is immediately available to the referring provider. More commonly, however, dermatology consultant notes and letters are typed or handwritten, and then faxed or sent by mail to the referring provider.

Personal communication between providers caring for the same patient is always conducive to quality care, but in teledermatology, it is arguably even more important to pick up the phone and call the referring provider from time to time to discuss a shared patient. Physicians like to know to whom they are referring their patients. Being separated geographically from the specialists they use can be a psychological barrier for referring providers and proactively nurturing these relationships will keep the referral lanes open and help to maintain access to quality dermatological care for patients in rural and underserved areas.

Conclusion

This discussion offers but a few of the challenges and opportunities facing practitioners of live-interactive teledermatology. Each clinical situation will be slightly different and present unique opportunities and challenges. Keeping an open mind and a willingness to tap into one's creative nature will promote a successful live-interactive teledermatology practice. Because of the challenges, it is sometimes tempting to consider live-interactive or hybrid teledermatology as being something less than the gold standard of in-person care. It is useful to keep in mind, however, that for many patients in remote areas, both geographically and logistically, care and treatment will be given via teledermatology or there will be no care at all.

Appendices

Appendix A: Sample patient questionnaire/survey form

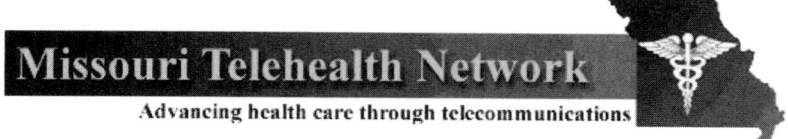

Patient questionnaire

Thank you for being a telehealth patient! It is very important to us to learn all we can about telehealth. We need your help. Please take a minute to complete this questionnaire. Your answers will be kept confidential.

Date: _____ Time: _____
Patient name: _____ Date of birth: _____

1 How far did you have to travel to get here? _____ miles (one way)

2 How far would you have to travel to see the telehealth provider in person? _____ miles (one way)
   [The *telehealth provider* is the out-of-town doctor or other health professional you saw on the TV.]

3 How would you have handled your health problem without telehealth?

   _____ Would not have received health care at this point. (Go to question #6)

   _____ Would have received health care in my own community. (Go to question #6)

   _____ Would have traveled out of town for health care.

4 What town would you have traveled to for your health care?
   _____

5 How many miles is it from your home (one way)? _____miles

6 Please circle the number that best shows your overall satisfaction with today's telehealth session.

1	2	3	4	5	6	7
Very dissatisfied	Dissatisfied	Somewhat dissatisfied	Neutral	Somewhat satisfied	Satisfied	Very satisfied

7 Please add any comments you have about telehealth or this project:

Thank you very much for your responses!

Appendix B: Sample teledermatology history intake form

Missouri Telehealth Network - Consultation Request Form

Site Name _____ Contact _____ Phone _____ Fax _____

✳ BEFORE appointment, fax COMPLETED form to MTN: (573) 882-5666 ✳

CONSULTATION INFORMATION

Patient Name:Last _____ First _____ MI ___ Appt Date &

Time _____

Nature of Request _____

Provider Seeking Consult _____ PCP Physician _____

Dx (if one was made) _____

History and Present Illness _____

_____

_____

Has the patient been seen at University of Missouri Health Care before?   YES   NO

PATIENT INFORMATION

Street Address _____

Mailing Address (if different) _____

City, State and Zip _____

Home phone (   )_____ Work phone (   )_____ Cell phone (

)_____

Occupation _____ Employer _____

DOB _____ SSN# _____

If under 18, name of parent/guardian _____

Sex: Male   Female   Race: White   Black   Hispanic   American

Indian   Asian   Other

Marital Status: Single   Married   Spouse/Guarantor Name _____

In case of emergency, whom do we contact? Name _____

Relationship _____

Address _____ Phone _____

INSURANCE INFORMATION

INSURANCE? (circle ALL that apply)   Self-Pay   Medicare   Medicaid   HMO   PATOS

POS/PPO   Commercial

Does this Insurance require a referral?   YES   NO

Ins Co Name _____   Ins Co Address _____

City _____ State _____ Zip _____ Ins Co Phone (

)_____

Subscriber's Name _____   Patient Relationship to

Subscriber _____

Subscriber's Gender: Male   Female   Subscriber's Date of Birth _____

Insurance Id # _____   Group # _____

Effective Date _____

Responsible Party's Name _____ SSN _____

Address of Responsible

Party _____

University
Hospital
University of Missouri Health Care

Patient Name _____

_____

Medical Record No _____

Appointment Date _____

Dermatology Clinic Patient Information Sheet

Site Name _____ Contact _____ Phone _____ Fax _____

❋ BEFORE appointment, fax COMPLETED form to Derm Clinic: (573)

884-0723 ❋

━━━━━━━━━━━━━━━━━━━━━━━━━━━━━━━━━━━━━━

Name _____ Date _____

Please circle any symptoms, sign, or conditions you are currently experiencing:

Fever	Nausea/vomiting	Mole changes	Itching	Skin rashes
Pregnancy sores	Diarrhea	New growth	Non-healing	
Tenderness	Other _____			

Past Medical History/Family History

Disease	Yourself	Family	Disease	Yourself	Family
Acne	_____	_____	High cholesterol	_____	_____
Asthma/hay fever	_____	_____	Kidney disease	_____	_____
Bleeding disorder	_____	_____	Joint replacement	_____	_____
Depression	_____	_____	Liver dz/Hepatitis	_____	_____
Diabetes	_____	_____	Psoriasis	_____	_____
Eczema	_____	_____	Recurrent yeast inf	_____	_____
Fever blister	_____	_____	Skin Cancer	_____	_____
Heart or renal transplant	_____	_____	Heart valve dz/Murmur	_____	_____

What is your occupation?_____ Do you smoke?   Yes   No

What outdoor activities do you enjoy? _____

Do you drink alcohol?   Yes   No   How often? _____

Do you wear sunscreen?   Yes   No   Have you ever used a tanning bed?   Yes   No

Have you ever had blistering sunburn?   Yes   No   Are you a student?   Yes   No

Are you planning a pregnancy?   Yes   No   Date of last menstrual period _____

Current medications including non-prescription, allergy and birth control: _____
_____
_____

━━━━━━━━━━━━━━━━━━━━━━━━━━━━━━━━━━━━━━

Preferred pharmacy _____ Pharmacy phone _____

Daytime phone _____ Evening/cell phone_____

Patient Signature _____ Date _____

Appendix C: Training requirements for a store-and-forward teledermatology consult manager

Requirement: Approximately 8 hr of initial training

1. Receive hands-on training on a digital camera (up to 2 hr).
2. Receive training on photographic techniques specific to teledermatology (Macro Imaging, Standards-based imaging protocol, Lighting, Hair imaging, etc). See appendix D (up to 3 hr).
3. Learn the basic terms used in clinical dermatology as it relates to four major characteristics of skin disease (up to 1 hr).
4. Learn to recognize the 10 most common skin conditions (classic-type only) to include seborrheic dermatitis, nevus, eczema, psoriasis, melanoma, basal cell carcinoma, and squamous cell carcinoma (up to 1 hr).
5. Receive hands-on training on the application to be used to enter consult data and upload images (up to 1 hr).
6. Receive training on consult flow for his or her organization to include the patient enrollment procedures, follow-up procedures, and exclusion criteria for teledermatology (up to 2 hr).
7. Receive training on how to prepare and set up room to take images of patients (use of background, lighting, etc.) (up to 1 hr).

Appendix D: Store-and-forward teledermatology imaging protocol

Imaging protocol (used with permission from TeleDerm Solutions)

1. Identify anatomic units based on location(s) of skin involvement.
2. Determine if complementary views are needed.
3. Take close-up images.

1 Anatomic unit

Determine the location(s) of the skin condition. Then determine what region(s) are involved and take the included standard view of the region(s) as listed below. Anatomic regions/units – standard views

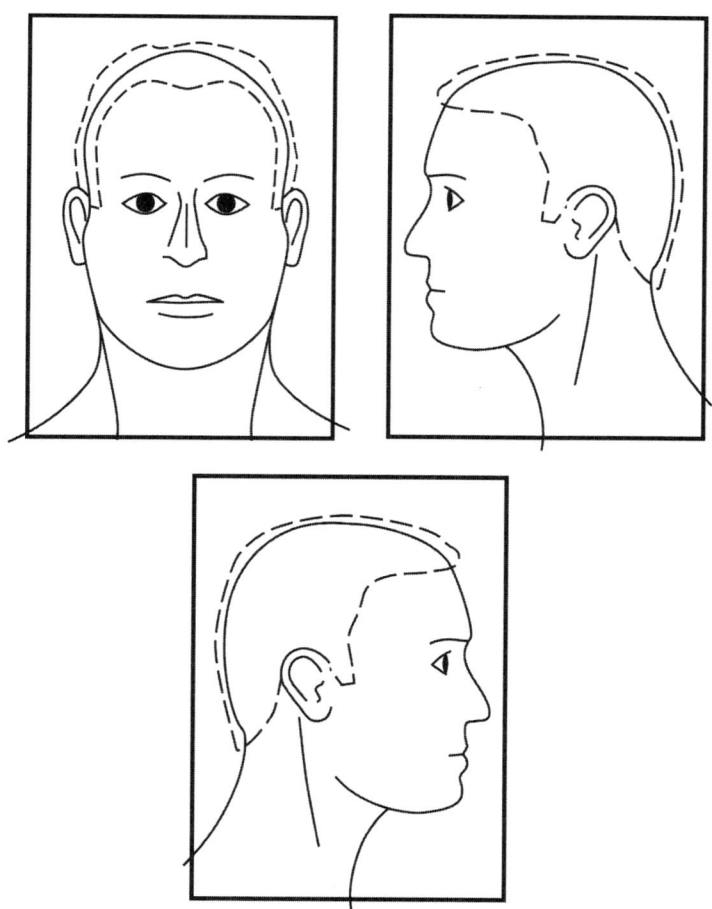

Face/neck standard set

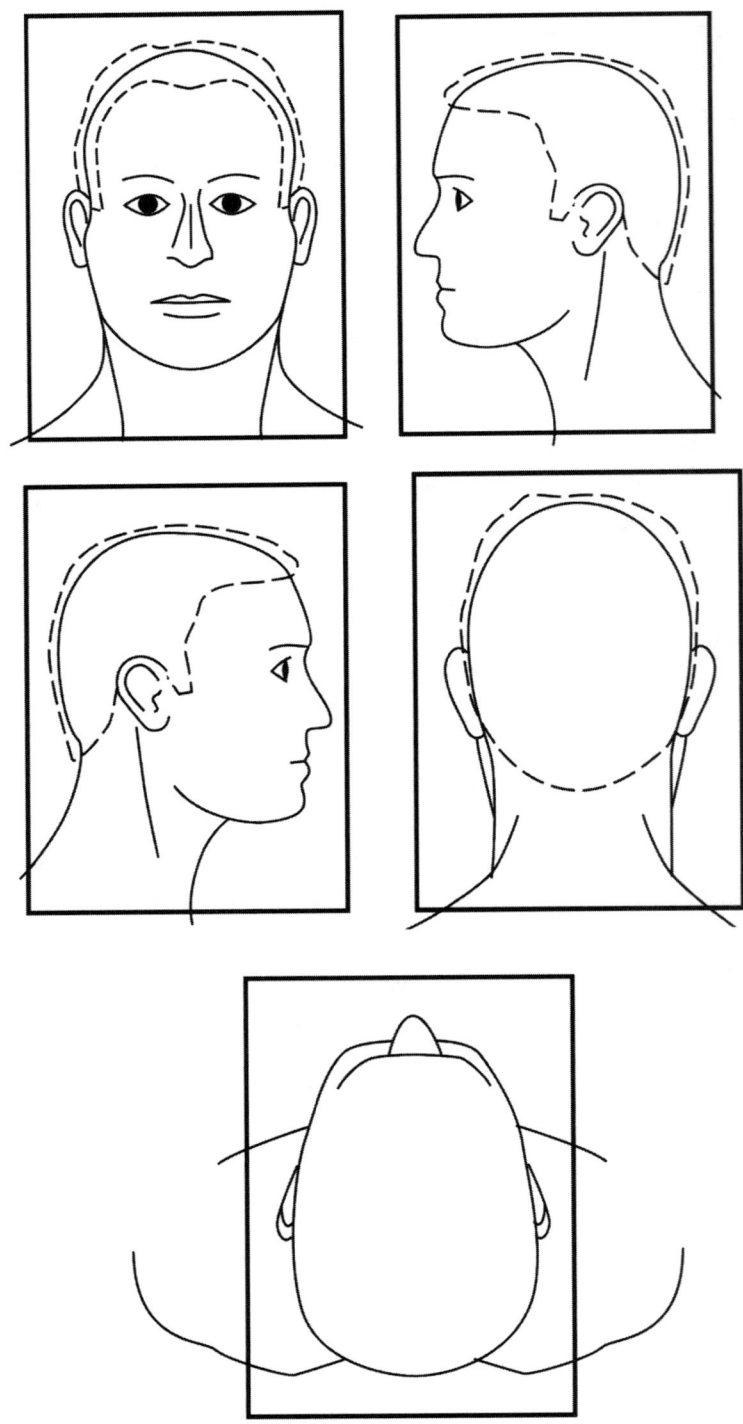

Scalp/hair standard set

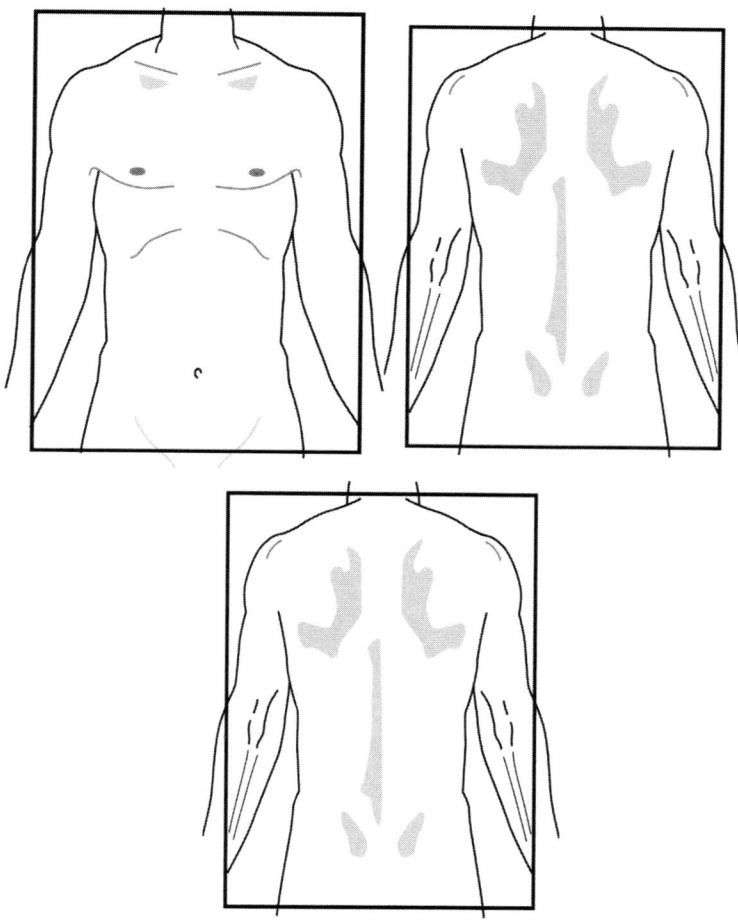

Trunk standard set

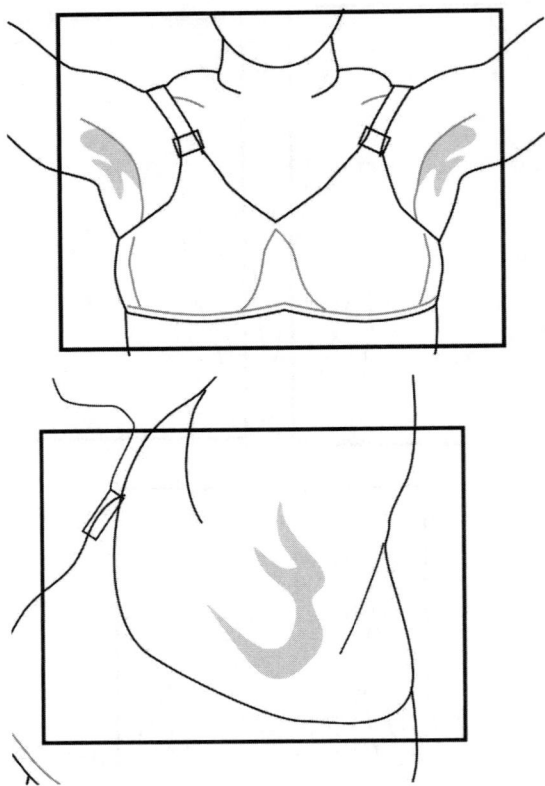

Axilla

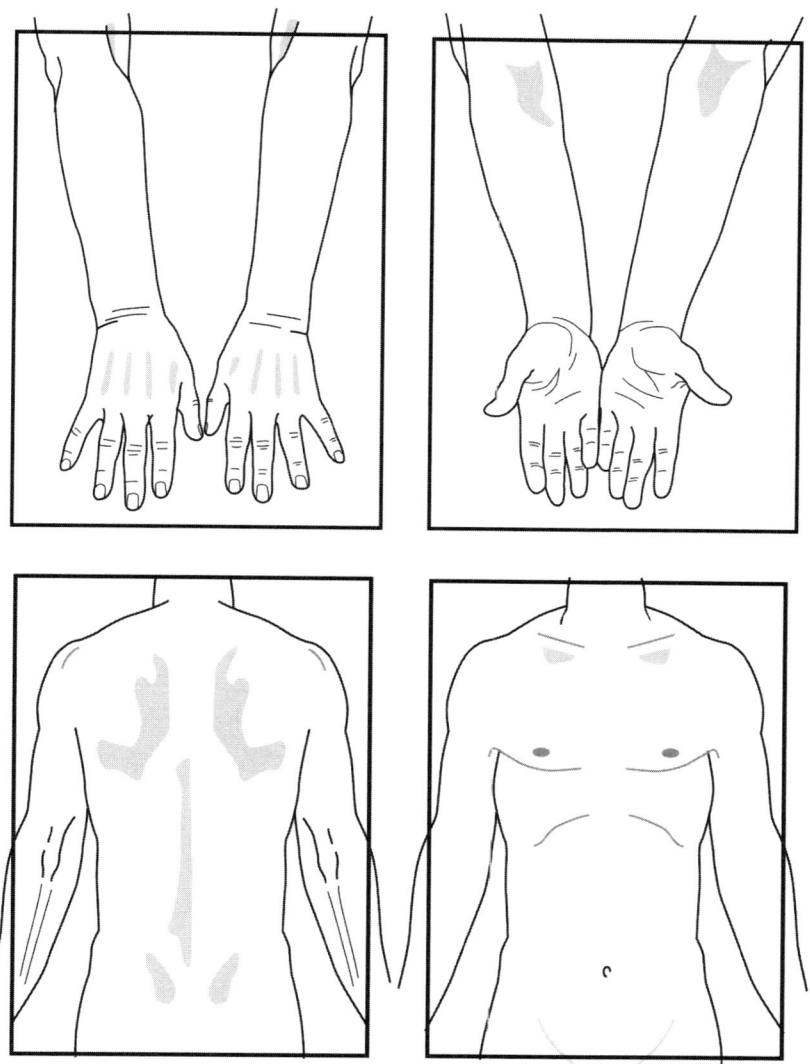

Arm standard set

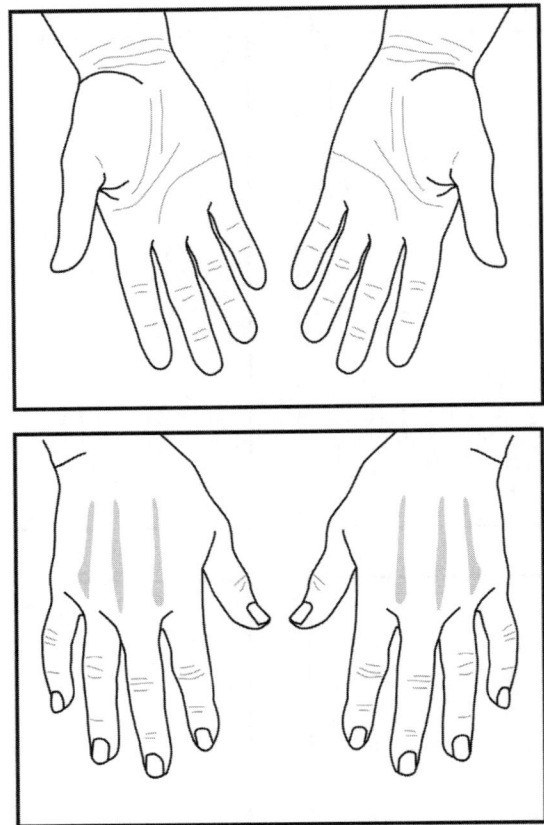

Hand standard set

Optional view (if lateral aspect of fingers are involved)

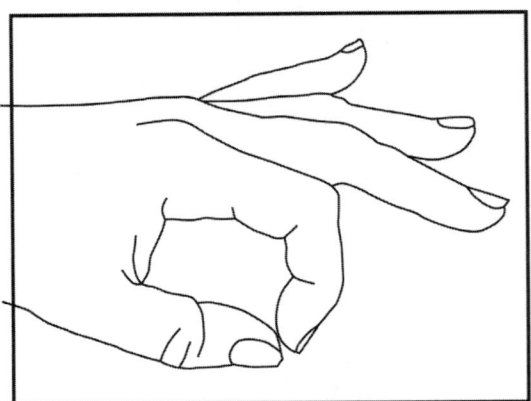

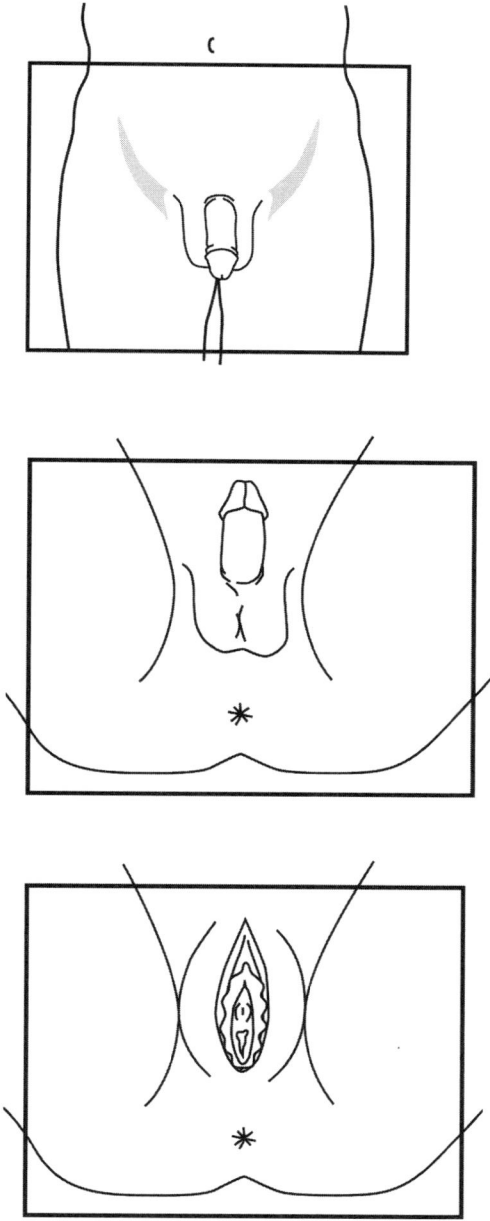

Groin/buttock standard set

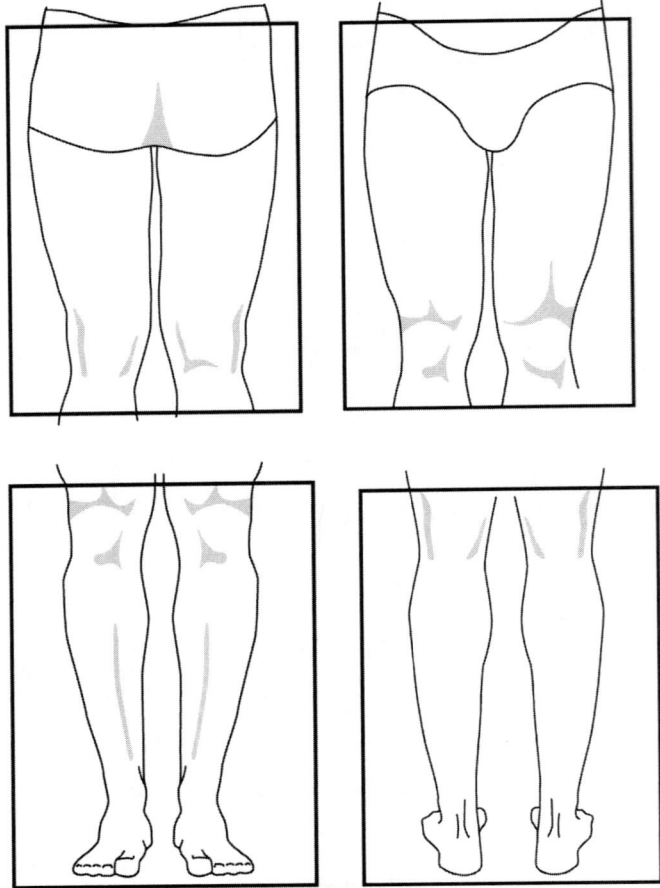

Leg standard set

Optional views: The images given below are optional and needed when the lesions are located predominantly on the medial or lateral aspect.

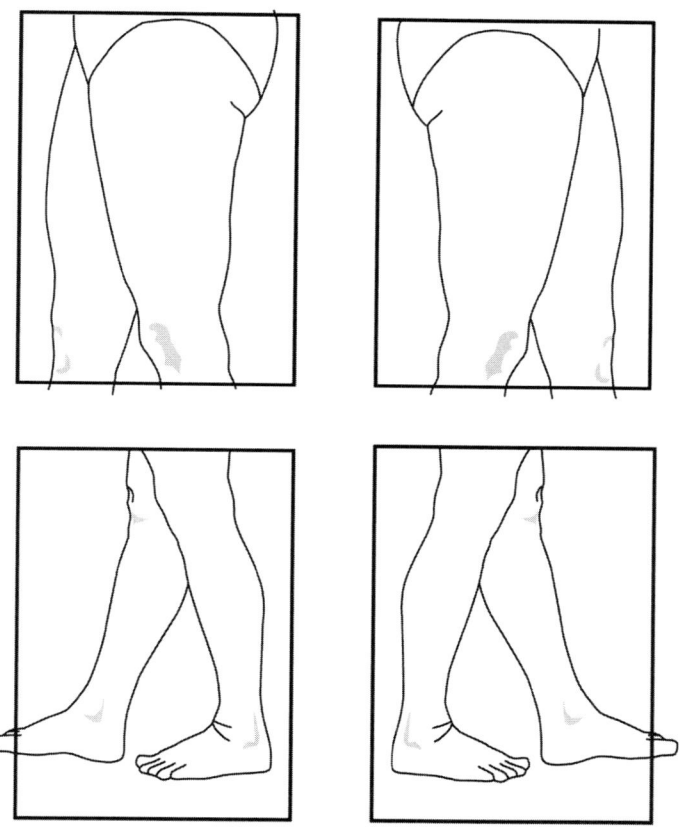

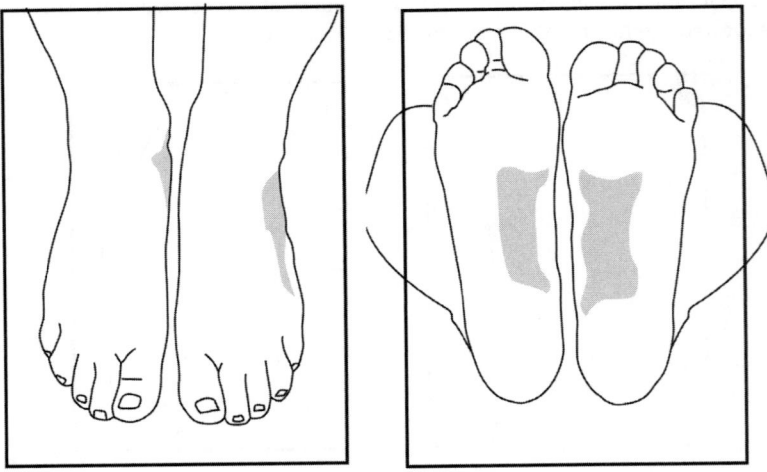

Feet standard set

2 Complementary sets

If the skin condition involves the listed locations (in column A), then take the listed complementary views (in column B) and document presence or absence of skin involvement (in column C).

(A) If involved	(B) Include	(C) Evaluate and document
Hands	Feet	Elbows/knees
Feet	Hands	Groin
Elbows	Knees	Scalp
Knees	Elbows	Scalp
Scalp	Face	Knees, elbows
Popliteal fossa	Antecubital fossa	Neck, face, hands
Antecubital fossa	Popliteal fossa	Neck, face, hands
Nail (any)	All nails	Oral mucosa
Groin	Buttocks	Hands and feet
Face (eyebrows, NLF)		Scalp
Oral mucosa		Genitals

Examples of common complementary sets:

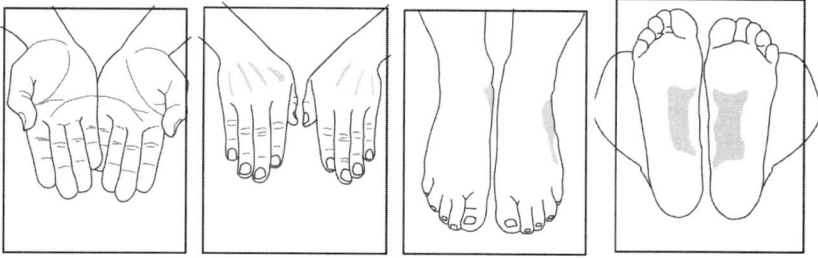

A Hands/feet

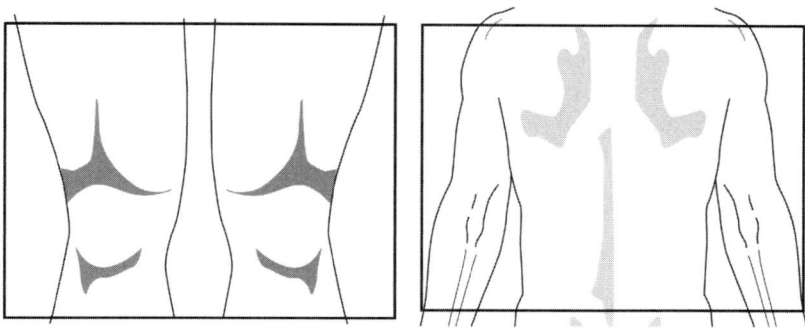

B Knees/elbows

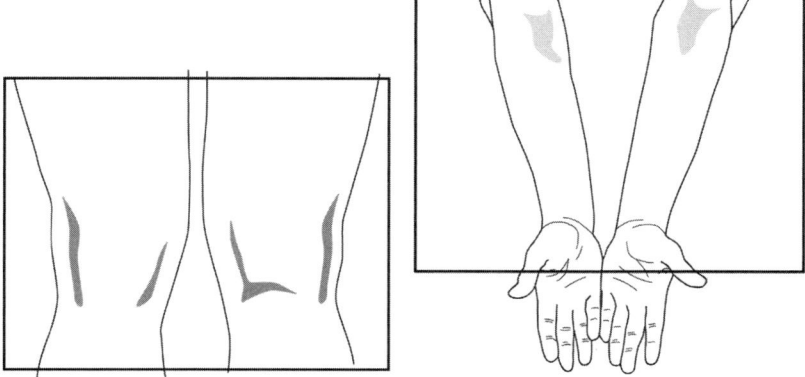

C Popliteal fossa/antecubital fossa

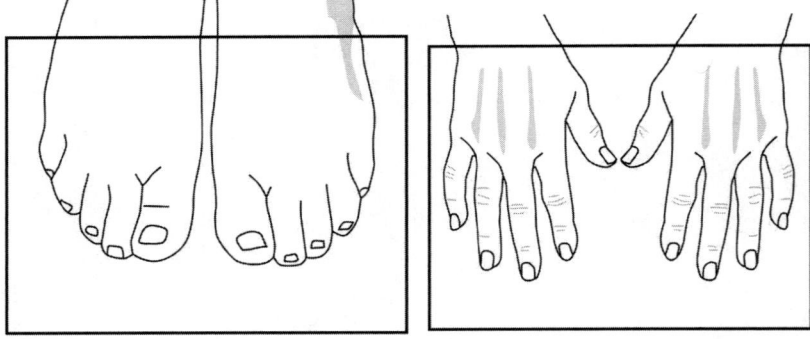

D Nails

3 Close ups

Examine the body for representative lesions and take one or more close ups as needed (more needed if there is more than one representative lesion). Also look for patterns/configurations (linear, grouped, annular, etc.) and consider obliques only if lesion height is subtle (lipoma, epidermal inclusion cyst). Do not get closer than 6–12" and attempt to standardize all close ups at a fixed distance (12" typically) and take the image perpendicular to the area of interest.

Appendix E: Sample technical protocol for real-time teledermatology

Missouri Telehealth Network
Advancing health care through telecommunications

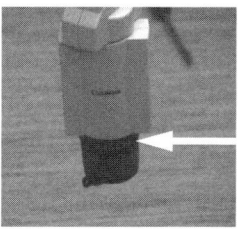

Figure 1

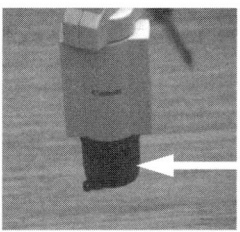

Figure 2

Canon Vizcam 1000

1. Turn on the power switch for the Vizcam, located on the right side of the base. The *tally lamp* will light. *(Note: The tally lamp is the small green light located at the front of the base of the Vizcam.)*
2. Select the Vizcam camera by using the Polycom remote control. Press the **NEAR** button followed immediately by the **2** button on the numeric keypad to select Camera 2.
3. Adjust lighting and focus. The black ring with numbers (Figure 1) on it adjusts the aperture (available light), and the brown ring (Figure 2) will adjust the focus. The recommended aperture setting is 2.8.

Using the vizcam 1000 for dermatology

1. This camera must be moved into position and stabilized in order for the dermatologist to receive the best quality image. Stabilization is best accomplished using a tripod, table, or cart. In no instance should this camera be handheld – it will produce an unacceptable level of motion artifacts for the dermatologist.
2. For very close work, it may be necessary to focus an additional light source on the subject. The vizcam does not have an independent light source, and depends on the available light in the room.

(continued)

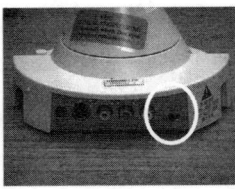

Figure 3

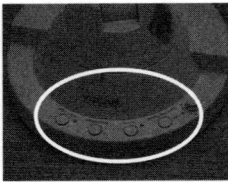

Figure 4

Troubleshooting suggestions

1. Be sure the lens cover has been removed from the camera.
2. Be sure the camera head is pointing at something besides a blank wall or tabletop.
3. The DC IN power cable on the Vizcam must be plugged into a power outlet.
4. SHUTTER SPEED selection switch on the base of the Vizcam should be set to 1/60 (Figure 3).
5. All LED indicators on the base of the Vizcam should default to the OFF (unlit) status (Figure 4). Press selector switches once to toggle off if necessary.

Updated April 12, 2002

Appendix F: Store-and-forward teledermatology protocol

Appropriate patient and type of consult

All patients are eligible for teleconsultation if they have been referred by their primary care physician for a skin condition. The referring provider makes the decision on whether to utilize teledermatology. However, a full body skin exam is not recommended at this time using store and forward. Rather, it is recommended that the referring provider does the skin exam and refer the patient if there are any questions or concerns about a specific lesion or lesions. If there is an urgent consult, the consult manager from the referring site should contact the specialist or telehealth coordinator.

Referral and scheduling process

Patients should ideally have their image and history obtained immediately after the referring provider decides on the consult. However, patient may be brought back for a separate visit later based on patient's convenience or resource available at the referring site.

Telehealth encounter procedure

ROOM PREPARATION

➠ Ensure that the examination room is clean and that the digital camera is in working order (including fully charged battery).
➠ Ensure that the necessary tables/chairs are available for both history intake and the standards-based imaging.

PATIENT PREPARATION

➠ Originating site telehealth coordinator will obtain the appropriate participation consent forms (if needed) immediately prior to the first telehealth consultation per patient. A copy of the consent form will be kept in patients chart, and the original kept in patient's chart/record.
➠ Site coordinator at patient site will explain to patients how telehealth consults take place, including that this system is confidential.
➠ Originating consult manager or other health-care professional responsible for taking the appropriate history (using a teledermatology consult worksheet) and confirming any information using patient's chart when available.

IMAGE CAPTURE

➠ Originating consult manager or other healthcare professional responsible for taking the appropriate images using the imaging protocol and reviewing the images prior to patient leaving the facility.

➠ originating consult manager will submit the consult online using a secure teleconsultation application.

PATIENT INSTRUCTIONS

Consult manager will tell the patient that he or she will be contacted within a week. Any face-to-face referrals will be arranged by the consult manager.

Teledermatology consult worksheet

The site consult manager may ask a sample of patients to complete the "patient questionnaire." Referring provider may complete the consult worksheet.

Report from teledermatologist

Teledermatologist will answer all consults within 3 business days of the consult submission. The consult will include at a minimum diagnosis, differential diagnosis, work-up/tests/management recommendations to include follow-up instructions.

If a dermatology resident answers the consult first, the consult must be reviewed before the consult report is sent back to the referring provider. Each consult report will be printed and given to the referring provider or made available electronically. The report should become part of the patient's medical record.

Appendix G: Real-time interactive teledermatology protocol

Telehealth dermatology encounter – MU Health Care

APPROPRIATE PATIENT AND TYPE OF CONSULT

For those patients who, in the opinion of their physician, can receive follow-up exams via the telehealth system or have been referred by their primary care physician for a condition appropriate to be seen by a specialist through the use of the telehealth system.

REFERRAL AND SCHEDULING PROCESS

Patients call the Patient Access and Referral Services (PARS) at 573-882-7000 or 800-882-9000.

TELEHEALTH ENCOUNTER PROCEDURE

Physicians may schedule a physician consult by calling 573-877-7197.

Preexamination

WRITTEN DOCUMENTS

➠ Once an appointment is obtained, either the patient, the referring physician, or the originating site telehealth coordinator will FAX to the hub provider site patient registration information to include name, address, phone numbers, SS#, DoB, current insurance, referring physician, prior diagnosis related to this consult, all current medications and doses, and any other pertinent information needed for the chart.

➠ Originating site telehealth coordinator will obtain the appropriate participation consent forms (adult or minor) immediately prior to the first telehealth consultation per patient. Additional consent forms are not required for subsequent visits, but consultations cannot proceed without a signed consent on file. A copy of the consent form will be kept in patients chart, and the original sent within 5 working days to the MTN office at

2401 Lemone Industrial Blvd.
DC345.00
Columbia, MO 65212.

ROOM PREPARATION

➠ To connect the telehealth system, MUHC initiates the call using the Polycom address book and the other site answers the call.

➠ Microphone(s) are highly sensitive and therefore the only consideration is placing the microphone(s) away from the monitor's speakers.

➠ Confirm that the Elmo and the Vizcam cameras at the patient site are working properly.

PATIENT PREPARATION

➠ Site coordinator at patient site will explain to patients participating in their first telehealth consult how telehealth consults take place, including that this system is confidential and only the healthcare professionals attending this consult and the patient can see and hear this session. Return patients should be reminded of this.

➠ Site coordinator or other healthcare professional at the patient site may take and record the patient's vital signs before the consult begins (weight, blood pressure, pulse, and respiratory rate).

➠ Originating site coordinator or other healthcare professional responsible for the patient will bring the patient's chart to the telehealth consultation in order to provide any needed information.

➠ Originating site coordinator or other healthcare professional responsible for the patient will stay with the patient during the telehealth consultation to operate the telehealth system, assist the patient as needed, to present any additional information the provider physician at the hub site may need, and take any orders given by provider physician at hub site.

Examination

EQUIPMENT

In addition to the basic videoconferencing system, a dermatology consult may include the use of the Elmo or the Canon Vizcam cameras to show patient characteristics and skin conditions. Cameras at both the physician and the patient sites should be set as per physician instructions.

ACTIVITIES

Interactive conversation with both patient and others (family, helper, etc.) present in the room at the patient site. Use the Elmo camera or Canon Vizcam camera to examine specific skin area(s).

Postexamination

PATIENT INSTRUCTIONS

Provider physician will tell patient if and when they are to schedule a return visit, either via telehealth or in person. The originating site coordinator or other healthcare professional responsible for the patient will note this to chart and coordinate the return visit with the dermatology department.

EVALUATION FORMS

The site coordinator may ask a sample of patients to complete the "patient questionnaire." Provider at hub site will be asked to complete "Office Staff" form. The site coordinator at the patient site will return all completed forms (fax or mail) within 5 working days to the MTN office at

2401 Lemone Industrial Blvd.
DC345.00,
Columbia MO 65212

Appendix H: Is teledermatology right for you? (private practice dermatologists)

INTRODUCTION

➠ Whether it is appropriate for your setting depends on multiple factors.

➠ Disciplined approach is needed to make a determination of appropriateness.

➠ Plenty of help is available.

STEP 1: WHAT PROBLEM ARE YOU TRYING TO SOLVE?

➠ Access
  - Distance (extend reach to rural areas)
  - Time (long wait time)
  - Population (Medicaid)

➠ Optimization of resources
  - Triage
  - Consult routing (procedure/accutane clinic)

➠ Life style
  - Flexible hours
    - Stay at home
    - Early retirement
  - Additional income

➠ Supervision
  - Remote satellite clinics
  - Nursing homes
  - In patients

➠ Shortage of dermatologists
  - Virtual staff

➠ Volunteer
  - International
  - National
    - Uninsured
  - Missions
  - HIV clinic
  - Disasters
    - Natural
    - Man-made

STEP 2: WHAT IS YOUR ECONOMIC OBJECTIVE?

➠ Cost neutral (outreach)

➠ Cost optimization: Decrease referrals to outside your network (University Health Plan)

⮞ Revenue: Demand from outside organization (University of Miami)
- VA
- HMO
- DoD

STEP 3: WHAT TYPE OF ORGANIZATION DO YOU BELONG TO?
⮞ Private practice
⮞ University
⮞ VA/DoD
⮞ HMO

STEP 4: WHERE ARE THE PATIENTS COMING FROM?

STEP 5: SELECT A BUSINESS MODEL
⮞ Primary revenue model
- Fee basis contract (per consult)
- Traditional reimbursement (Medicaid/Medicare/third-party billing)
- Grant (uninsured)
⮞ Secondary revenue model
- Referral for specialty care
  ▪ Cosmetic/laser
  ▪ Moh's
- Non derm referrals (international model)
⮞ Optimization model (savings from various sources)
- Decreased unnecessary referrals (teleconsultation)
- PCMs manage higher percentage of skin conditions
- Lower total costs (more efficient utilization)
- Higher productivity (triage)
⮞ Outreach model
- Volunteer
- National disaster response
- Teaching/education (HIV)
- Grants/non-profit
⮞ Supervision model
- Resident
- NP/PA
⮞ Other
- Virtual inpatient/nursing home visit

STEP 6: SELECT MODALITY/TECHNOLOGY
⮞ Modality
- Telecare (direct patient care)
- Teleconsultation (provider to provider)
- Teletriage (triage only)

⮕ Technology
  - VTC (education/teaching but low volume)
  - S&F (scalability – high volume)
  - Hybrid

STEP 7: REFERRAL SITE CHECKLIST
⮕ Technical capability
  - Equipment
  - Bandwidth
  - Human resources
  - Dedicated technician available
  - Part time availability
  - Existing procedures/policy
  - Triage
  - Referral process
  - Follow up
  - Path specimen management
  - Capability
  - Procedures (shave biopsy/punch biopsy)
  - Dermatology follow up (local dermatologist access)
  - Derm supply
  - Cryotherapy

STEP 8: CONSULTING SITE/CAPACITY
⮕ Technical capability
  - Equipment (VTC, PC)
  - Bandwidth (POTS, cable, DSL)
  - Human resources (technical support)
⮕ Professional capability
  - Turnaround requirement
  - Moh's, laser, cosmetic
  - Inclusion and exclusion
⮕ Dermatology capacity
  - Blocked time available (Mon AM)
  - Time available after hours
  - Integrated with clinic
  - Free time while away from work
    - Relationship with referring providers
    - Liability insurance (telemedicine)
    - Billing: registered/credentialed with payers
    - State-specific laws
⮕ Supervision
⮕ Licensure

STEP 9: DETERMINE IF THIS IS ECONOMICALLY FEASIBLE.

⟶ Revenue
- Approximately $25–100 per consult
- Many are using normal consulting codes (9924x/9927x)
- Negotiable in some cases
- Average volume: 8–20 consults/hr
- Estimate demand/volume

⟶ Cost (overhead) for consultants – estimate only
- Varies based on technology used
- Technology selection should be based on need

⟶ S&F
- Hardware (PC < $1k)
- Software (application) varies $100–200 per month
- Bandwidth ($40 per month)

⟶ VTC
- Hardware ($1–5k)
- Bandwidth ($100–200 per month)

⟶ Hybrid
- Hardware (<$1k)
- Software application varies $100–200 per month
- Bandwidth ($40–200 per month)
- Administrative costs
- Liability insurance
- Other

STEP 10. IMPLEMENTATION STEP (ASSUMING THAT YOU HAVE GONE THROUGH THE STEPS ABOVE AND HAVE DECIDED THAT TELEDERMATOLOGY IS FEASIBLE FOR YOU, THE NEXT STEP IS TO GET HELP)

- Most difficult step
- Plenty of help available
- ATA Teledermatology SIG
- AAD Telemedicine Taskforce
- Consultants
- Addition steps remaining
- Training
- Software/hardware for referral sites
- Billing
- Coordination

SUMMARY

- Objectives/what problem are you trying to solve?
- What is your availability/capacity?

- Who is your customer/is there a real demand?
- Determine business model?
- What is the best technology?
- Does this make economic sense?
- Get some help.

Index